T0032682

DAY TO DAY
LIVING WITH
DEMENTIA

A MAYO CLINIC GUIDE
FOR OFFERING
CARE AND SUPPORT

Angela M. Lunde, M.A.

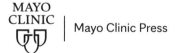

MAYO
CLINIC

Mayo Clinic Press

MAYO CLINIC

Medical Editor | Angela M. Lunde, M.A.

Publisher | Daniel J. Harke

Editor in Chief | Nina E. Wiener

Senior Editor | Karen R. Wallevand

Managing Editor | Stephanie K. Vaughan

Art Director | Stewart J. Koski

Illustration, Photography and Production | Amanda J. Knapp

Editorial Research Librarians | Abbie Y. Brown, Anthony J. Cook, Edward (Eddy) S. Morrow Jr., Erika A. Riggin, Katherine (Katie) J. Warner

Contributors | Laura M. Waxman; Ericka E. Tung, M.D., M.P.H.; Jodi L. Melius, R.N.

Additional contributors | Kirkus Media LLC, Steve Rath

Image Credits | All photographs and illustrations are copyright of MFMER.

Published by Mayo Clinic Press

©2022 Mayo Foundation for Medical Education and Research (MFMER)

MAYO, MAYO CLINIC and the Mayo triple-shield logo are marks of Mayo Foundation for Medical Education and Research. All rights reserved. No part of this book may be reproduced, stored in a retrieval system, or transmitted, in any form or by any means, electronic, mechanical, photocopying, recording or otherwise, without the prior written permission of the publisher.

The information in this book is true and complete to the best of our knowledge. This book is intended only as an informative guide for those wishing to learn more about health issues. It is not intended to replace, countermand or conflict with advice given to you by your own physician. The ultimate decision concerning your care should be made between you and your doctor. Information in this book is offered with no guarantees. The author and publisher disclaim all liability in connection with the use of this book.

For bulk sales to employers, member groups and health-related companies, contact Mayo Clinic, 200 First St. SW, Rochester, MN 55905 or email SpecialSalesMayoBooks@mayo.edu.

When you purchase Mayo Clinic newsletters and books, proceeds are used to further medical education and research at Mayo Clinic. You not only get the answers to your questions on health, you become part of the solution.

ISBN 978-1-945564-23-9

Library of Congress Control Number: 2022932928

Printed in the United States of America

Table of Contents

Foreword

Frequently, I sit with patients and families coping with dementia. For the newly diagnosed, I discuss the realities of the disease that's causing the dementia and the course it may take. As carefully as I can, I share what they may see in the weeks, months and years ahead. Then, over time, I care for them and their families as the disease progresses and transforms the person with dementia in ways that are often hard to accept and cope with.

Despite dementia's many changes and challenges, there's one constant: the care partner. Offering an unwavering presence, care partners seek to understand, care for and guide those living with dementia, helping them stay safe, live with dignity and maintain a quality life. Without supportive care partners, my work as a doctor would be impossible. As health care professionals, we honor you for all that you're doing, every single day, for always being there and for helping us provide care. The time and energy you invest in supporting someone with dementia does not go unnoticed.

I'll say that again, in another way for emphasis: We as doctors cannot optimally care for people living with dementia without you, the care partner, and the invaluable work you do. What you're doing is love.

And yet, day after day, I see care partners struggle. I see sadness. Loneliness. Frustration. Despair. There are many real — and often hard — emotions that care partners experience along the dementia journey. Know that your voices and your feelings are being heard.

No matter what challenges you're facing in this moment, you're not alone. Legions of people have walked this path before you. In addition, your health care team is at the ready, prepared to answer questions and eager to help you find the support you need, whether it's respite, resources or someone to talk to. Know that we are here for you.

This book provides just the kind of support that health care providers strive to offer in their offices every day. As you read the following pages, you will find validation for many of the emotions caregivers express, including guilt and burnout. Even more important, I hope that in this book you feel treated as the valuable human being that you are — and that, ultimately, you're more able to allow yourself grace, no matter where in the dementia journey you find yourself.

One of the most important things you can do as a caregiver is to take a step back for a moment and assess your resources, assemble your team and create a plan that helps you navigate day-to-day living with dementia. This book will help you do just that; use what you learn in the chapters of this book to guide you and shape the ongoing conversations you have with your health care team.

You are not alone. No matter what, you have support — and this book is one way we can ensure that.

Dr. Eseosa T. Ighodaro
Department of Neurology, Mayo Clinic

Preface

Over the past two decades, I've met thousands of women and men who find themselves in a new role called caregiver, or care partner. Some of them find the strength, resilience and resources to overcome many of the extraordinary challenges they face. For most, however, this is not the case, and they feel alone, overwhelmed and unprepared for this new role. Without a doubt, the dementia caregiving experience is emotionally volatile, is physically exhausting and can last a long time.

There is no one right way to provide care and support to a person living with dementia, and there are no easy answers. My hope is that this book helps shape an attitude and an approach to dementia care, and self-care, that can help in the months and years ahead. In addition, this book is a practical guide that addresses the questions and concerns I hear from care partners on topics such as understanding and navigating changes in behavior, adjusting communication, planning ahead and working with health care professionals.

Caregivers are one of the most treasured resources in our society; may we walk alongside them with a listening ear, nonjudging presence and unconditional support.

Angela M. Lunde, M.A.

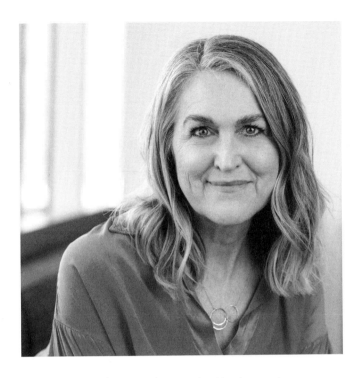

Angela M. Lunde, M.A., has worked in dementia care, education and research for over 20 years as an associate in neurology in the Mayo Clinic Alzheimer's Disease Research Center. Ms. Lunde is involved in numerous partnerships focused on reducing stigma and supporting the inclusion and voice of people living with dementia. Her interests are focused on understanding the experience of living with dementia and the caregiving role. Her research and innovations center on addressing the emotional health and psychosocial needs of care partners and family systems to recognize greater potential for well-being. Ms. Lunde is co-medical editor of *Mayo Clinic on Alzheimer's Disease and Other Dementias*, has authored published peer-reviewed articles, has written numerous articles and book chapters, and has maintained an expert blog on dementia caregiving for more than a decade.

1

Adjusting to a diagnosis

Hearing the word *dementia* in a medical office can make you feel as if your whole world has changed drastically. Whether the diagnosis applies to you or to a loved one, simply hearing the word can come as a shock.

Leading up to this moment, it may have been hard enough to acknowledge your concerns, let alone bring them to a doctor's attention. After all, the onset of dementia is often gradual, so it's easy to pass off symptoms as a typical part of getting older.

Maybe you were hoping to hear something else — perhaps that forgetfulness and confusion were due to aging or that the symptoms would disappear with a change in medication. You may be flooded with disbelief. It's hard to imagine something like this happening to you or someone close to you.

Plus, the word *dementia* can stir up many commonly held beliefs, many of which aren't true. You may think, *There's nothing that can be done, My life is over, I'm going to be completely dependent on others for the rest of my life.* These are strong emotions to work through.

As you start to mull over a dementia diagnosis and what it means for you, use the information on the following pages to begin coming to terms with what comes next. This chapter offers guidance to help you adjust to and live well with a dementia diagnosis, whether you're the one who's received it or you're supporting someone who's been diagnosed with it.

EFFECTS ON THE PERSON DIAGNOSED WITH DEMENTIA

A dementia diagnosis is life altering. It means coming to terms with changes that, over time, cause increased challenges with memory and thinking, as well as language, physical abilities and emotions.

No matter what you're feeling, you're not alone. There's no right or wrong way to feel.

Some people struggle to accept the news and deny that they have dementia. It may come as a shock that symptoms aren't related to typical aging. Others have trouble understanding that they have dementia. They may lack insight about their impairment. The medical term for this is *anosognosia*. When someone lacks awareness of functional limitations, it can lead to risky behaviors, like driving when it's no longer safe to do so.

And finally, others say they felt prepared to hear the news, given the symptoms they'd been experiencing.

For some, a diagnosis offers a sense of relief. Many people find themselves feeling several different emotions all at once.

If you've been diagnosed with dementia, you may worry about not being able to do the things you've always done, and about becoming dependent on others or a burden. You may be concerned about what others will think of you. How will family, friends and others who know you react when they hear the news? Will they think of you differently, treat you differently or stop coming around altogether?

You may fear that you'll no longer be seen as a person with talents, strengths and abilities, and that instead, you'll be seen only as a person with dementia. You may feel sadness and a sense of loss, uncertain about your hopes and plans for the future. All these thoughts and concerns are understandable and common reactions.

WHAT IT MEANS TO HAVE LIMITED INSIGHT

Limited insight is when people lack full understanding about their cognitive impairment. It's often related to the type of dementia a person has or to the area of the brain that's affected. In some types of dementia, like frontotemporal degeneration, limited insight is common. In other types of dementia, like posterior cortical atrophy, limited insight is rare. Loss of insight tends to be linked to shrinkage (atrophy) in the right hemisphere of the brain.

Accepting a dementia diagnosis takes time, but it is a pathway toward taking positive action and restoring a sense of well-being.

After the initial shock and other strong feelings have settled a little, a diagnosis can often be viewed in a more positive light. The person who's been diagnosed and the person's family now know what they're dealing with and can start to take action and plan accordingly. In some ways, a diagnosis may even be a relief.

Just as there's no right or wrong way to feel about a dementia diagnosis, every person's path to accepting and living with it is different. Here's more on the many feelings family members may experience.

EFFECTS ON THE FAMILY

Family members often play a key role in recognizing symptoms that lead to a diagnosis. They're usually the ones who first notice the memory or other thinking changes, disorientation, changes in mood and sometimes personality. Family members often initiate a doctor visit out of concern that something's wrong. They may also have to help provide information on the diagnosis if the loved one doesn't completely understand it or is in a state of shock or denial.

There's generally a lag between the time family members first start to notice worrisome symptoms and when an appointment with a doctor is scheduled. The delay may be due to confusion about what are typical age-related changes and what are more serious developments. Often, the delay is a part of the process — the gradual realization that symptoms aren't getting any better and may be getting worse.

Denial can be the earliest and strongest emotion that family members feel. It's an understandable response to a difficult situation — as family members become aware that a loved one may have an incurable disorder, they worry about what the future holds and their ability to cope. Denial is a common response to uncertainty.

Sometimes, often before a dementia diagnosis, family members experience anger. Emotions like fear and

A POSITIVE OUTLOOK IS POSSIBLE

In a study of people diagnosed with dementia, about 1 in 3 said that focusing on what they could do and on the benefits of receiving a diagnosis allowed them to maintain a positive outlook.

For many, this focus involves making adjustments and accepting help. People interviewed for the study shared the following:

- It helps to accept that some things may need to be done differently — but that they still can be done. When reading a book, for instance, it may help to write down character names to remember them later.
- Making lists of things to remember is helpful.
- Reaching out to others who will support you can help you adjust to the news of a dementia diagnosis. Talk with someone you trust about what you're feeling.
- Reach out to others in practical ways too. For example, making a to-do list for the day and having someone review it can be helpful.

anxiety are often mixed in. They may think, *If only she would try harder*, *If only he would pay attention* or *I wish he'd listened to what I said*. These emotions are all natural to feel leading up to a diagnosis.

Often, and over time, a diagnosis offers a sense of relief. For example, the person with the diagnosis and family members can understand why the person's memory has been so unreliable or why there have been changes in mood.

At the same time, a diagnosis can lead to feelings of guilt as family members realize that behaviors that made them feel angry are due to a disease and are not the fault of the person.

It's important to forgive yourself when feelings of guilt arise. Getting angry or frustrated over things you didn't fully understand at the time is understandable. The good news is that with a diagnosis, you can move forward with understanding and empathy.

Even with a diagnosis , the road from denial to acceptance isn't a straight path. The person receiving the diagnosis, family members and friends may find themselves at different places along the journey at different times. Everyone will work through their feelings and adjust emotionally to the changes at their own pace. Each person's path is unique.

If you ever feel like you're the only one in this situation, remember that you're never alone. Millions of people around the world are living with the impact of Alzheimer's disease and other dementias. Millions more are in a supportive role. The first, and sometimes most difficult, step is accepting the diagnosis and adjusting to a new reality.

Talking to children

Adults may choose to shield young children from the knowledge that a family member has dementia. But children generally recognize when something is wrong. Your loved one's behavior may seem confusing, especially if the children don't understand why such behavior is occurring.

Here are ways to offer simple, honest answers to several questions children commonly ask.

- *Question:* What's wrong with Grandma?
  Explain that just as children can get sick, adults sometimes get an illness that causes them to act differently and to forget things. You may add that they might look like the same people on the outside, but their brains are changing on the inside.

- *Question:* Doesn't Grandpa love me anymore?
  Your child might feel rejected if the person with dementia no longer recognizes him or her. Remind your child that the disease makes it hard to remember things — but the person can still feel your child's love.

RANGE OF EMOTIONS

A diagnosis of Alzheimer's disease or another cause of dementia may trigger many moods and emotions. Disbelief, anger, shock, sadness, fear, devastation, relief, loss, embarrassment and numbness are all common. If you feel any one — or many — of these emotions, you're not alone.

- *Question:* Is it my fault?
  If the person with dementia accuses your child of wrongdoing — like stealing a belonging — your child might get upset.

  Explain that the person with dementia is confused. You might explain that it's best not to disagree with this person because it could make the person upset or frustrated.

- *Question:* Will other family members get Alzheimer's?
  Reassure your child that dementia isn't contagious. You might explain to an older child that just because a relative has dementia, it doesn't mean that every family member will get the disease.

- *Question:* What will happen next?
  If you'll be caring for the person who has dementia in your home, talk to your child about changes in your family's routine. Explain that the person will have good days and bad days.

If your child has trouble talking about the situation or withdraws from the person with dementia, open a conversation. Ask what changes your child has noticed. This might lead to a talk about your child's feelings and worries.

Tell your child it's OK to feel nervous, sad or angry. You might tell your child you feel that way sometimes too. To boost your child's understanding, seek out websites, books or videos on the disease.

A child may express emotions in indirect ways, like complaining of headaches or other physical problems. Your child might feel awkward around the person with dementia.

If the person with dementia is living in your home, your child may not feel comfortable inviting friends to the house or may look for ways to spend more time away from home. If you notice these behaviors, gently point out what you've seen — and offer your child comfort and support. Listen to your child's concerns.

NEXT STEPS

A diagnosis of dementia doesn't signal the end of living. On the contrary, a diagnosis can point you toward information, support, resources, treatments, clinical trials and services that can help. For the person living with dementia, one of the most important first steps after a diagnosis is to recognize that you have preserved strengths and abilities not affected by the disease and that there are many things you can do to continue to live a full life.

Here are several steps to take after a dementia diagnosis has been made. You'll gain more in-depth information later in this book.

Continue living your prediagnosis life as much as possible

Receiving a dementia diagnosis doesn't make you any different from who you were the day before the diagnosis. On the contrary, you are still the same person. One of the best things you can do after being diagnosed is to continue living your life as fully as you can. Very few people are diagnosed in the late stages of the disease, so there's a lot of living still to do. Staying engaged in life and doing things that keep you mentally and physically active are important.

Participate in support groups

People in the early stages of dementia often withdraw from friendships and social groups they once enjoyed because they're afraid that they'll make a mistake or embarrass themselves in some way.

But a diagnosis doesn't mean that socializing and friendships are less important now than they were before. In fact, being with others can improve overall well-being and increase a person's ability to adapt to the life changes that are occurring. The same is true for care partners.

This is where support groups for people with dementia and their care partners can help. A common theme echoed among support group participants is how valuable it is to be with others in similar situations who truly understand what they're going through.

Support groups can vary in their makeup and activities. Look for one that meets your needs. For example, some groups for people living with dementia gather in restaurants, cafés or museums. Other groups offer dementia-friendly activities, such as walking groups, volunteer programs or yoga designed for people with physical or cognitive impairments. The important thing is to find a group or an activity that allows you to feel comfortable sharing, growing and adapting.

Consider enrolling in research programs and clinical trials

The only way to develop new treatments or effective prevention efforts against dementia is through research and clinical trials with human volunteers. Participants at all stages and representing all aspects of dementia — including those who have dementia, care partners and even healthy individuals — are urgently needed. While every clinical trial has some risks, and it's important to understand those risks, there are many benefits as well.

Participating in research programs or a clinical trial can offer valuable support. At the same time, by taking an active role in dementia research, you can help future generations who might one day benefit from the results.

WORKPLACE TRANSITIONS

Life doesn't end with a dementia diagnosis. Although adjustments may be needed, many people with dementia can continue to live satisfying, active lives. This brings up a concern for many people diagnosed with dementia: Can I still work?

Whether or not to keep working — and what adjustments may be needed — are best evaluated on a case-by-case basis. Sometimes a team of experts, including a professional who specializes in occupational medicine, can help navigate these situations. In some cases, people with dementia can continue to work with some accommodations or in a different capacity.

As a first step, talk to your doctor about your symptoms and how they may affect your ability to work. This is a conversation you'll likely need to have on an ongoing basis as symptoms change over time.

Dementia is progressive, which means its symptoms gradually worsen over time. Most people living with dementia will need to transition out of the workforce

Find links to more information about clinical trials in the Resources section of this book.

Learn about treatment options

After receiving a diagnosis, you may feel that since no cure exists for dementia, there's no point in taking any

---

if they're not already retired. Your employer may offer benefits that can help, including an employee assistance program, which may include referrals, counseling and other assistance. Short-term disability and long-term disability are other possible benefits that may help during the transition. Social Security benefits are another possible option. Learn more in the Resources section of this book.

Transitioning out of the workforce can bring about feelings of uncertainty around identity and purpose. It's not uncommon for people with dementia to ask questions like, *What now? Who am I?* as they search for a new sense of identity and purpose. One way to address these questions is to explore skills you already have or take on activities that offer a fresh sense of purpose. You may look into opportunities that make use of your preserved strengths, interests and talents. If there are new activities you've always wanted to try, this may be the time to explore them. Connecting with others living with dementia may be another option.

medicine for it. But the diseases that cause dementia are often gradual in nature, and some medications may help slow the progression, while others can treat specific symptoms. In addition, services like counseling, occupational therapy, physical therapy and speech therapy can help preserve independence and improve quality of life.

HOW TO TALK ABOUT THE DIAGNOSIS

If you've been diagnosed with dementia, you may wonder when and how to share the news. It can be a difficult topic to discuss with others.

A big factor is your own personality and how comfortable you feel talking about personal issues with various people. Some people are likely to share the diagnosis with only a few close relatives and friends. Others may be much more open about their experience with dementia.

Wait until you feel ready to communicate with family and friends. You don't have to tell everyone at once. Come up with a list of people you need or want to tell first and a few brief talking points. If other family members have been through the diagnosis process with you, they can help. As you become more comfortable communicating the information, you can decide if there are others you want to tell. Or entrust a few reliable family members and friends with the task of sharing the news. What's most important is for you to feel comfortable and able to move forward with positive support.

Reactions may vary. Some are quick to provide support and offers of help. These are people who will be sensitive to your needs and want you to educate them about your condition. They're the ones who will respect you unconditionally, recognize your strengths and not make assumptions based on your diagnosis. They are also the ones who will laugh with you when you need a dose of humor. At times, relatives and friends you least expect become the most supportive.

But some people in your life may be unable to handle the news or confront their fears of what lies ahead for you. They may steer clear of any conversation about your health or avoid seeing you. Still others may say things that you feel are dismissive or insensitive. Try not to judge these people; they're handling the news in their own way. Over time, some may reach back out and find ways to be supportive.

Changes in relationships are common when a serious illness is diagnosed. Learning to accept these changes and leaning on stable relationships and friendships can help lessen some of the stress you may be feeling. If you're living with dementia, one of the most important things you can do is to talk about it. Let family, friends and others in your community know how they can support you. Assure them that you are still the same person you were before receiving the diagnosis but that you may need some help from time to time. This can help put others at ease and help you stay engaged and focused on the things that support your independence.

In addition, talking about dementia increases understanding and lessens fear, which can help reduce the stigma that often accompanies it.

Talking tips for care partners

Care partners often wonder whom to tell about the diagnosis and when to tell them. A person diagnosed

WHEN TO STOP DRIVING

Safe driving requires attention, concentration and the ability to follow particular steps and rules. It also requires the ability to make quick and appropriate decisions. For people with dementia, these skills can weaken over time. Eventually, driving will not be an option.

Even people with mild dementia are at a much greater risk of unsafe driving compared with people of the same age without dementia. The American Academy of Neurology recommends that people with mild dementia strongly consider discontinuing driving. With dementia, strengths and weaknesses vary from person to person, so it's important to talk about driving safety with a doctor or another professional as soon as possible.

Signs of unsafe driving include:
- Getting lost when driving to familiar places.
- Not staying in the lane.
- Confusing the brake and gas pedals.
- Failing to observe traffic signs.
- Making slow or poor decisions.
- Hitting the curb while driving.
- Driving too slowly or speeding.
- Becoming angry or confused while driving.
- Getting into an accident or getting a ticket.

People with mild dementia who are still able to drive safely may be able to drive for some time. If the person with dementia would still like to drive and it seems to be safe to do so, a roadside driving evaluation is strongly recommended. During this test, an occupational therapist or another driving expert evaluates the person's ability to drive and offers strategies for driving safely, as well as a plan for when and how to reduce or stop driving.

While giving up driving isn't a big issue for some people, for others, it's much more difficult. This is especially true for people with dementia who may lack insight into their limitations. In these cases, these strategies for care partners can help ease the situation, especially in cases of anger and resistance.

- Be patient but firm. With understanding and empathy, acknowledge how difficult this change likely is. At the same time, emphasize that not driving is a responsible choice to make.
- Enlist the help and support of your doctor. A message to discontinue driving coming from a medical professional may be better accepted than one from a family member. If not, at least the doctor can take the heat rather than a family member.
- If needed, ask someone that the person with dementia respects to reinforce the reasons why not driving is the best choice to make.
- Taking away car keys and even selling the car may be needed in some situations.

No matter the approach, it's important to make sure that the person with dementia continues to have a safe, reliable form of transportation.

with dementia may be afraid to feel "under the micro-scope" as people watch closely for signs of illness. You may be torn between protecting your loved one's privacy and sharing parts of the emotional roller coaster you're on.

As a first step, talk to the person diagnosed with dementia. It's important, first and foremost, to respect the privacy of someone who's been diagnosed with dementia. If the person with dementia is OK sharing the diagnosis with others, the next step is to decide how to share the news and determine whom to tell.

When sharing the diagnosis with others, explain the disease and its effects. It may help to share that demen-tia involves a disease that causes brain cells to degener-ate and die and that this causes a decline in memory and mental function. You may also explain what symptoms the person with dementia has now and the symptoms the person may have as the disease progresses. This is where educational materials from organizations like the Alzheimer's Association, the Lewy Body Dementia Association or other organizations can be helpful. They can help explain a disease, its effects and its symptoms. The Resources section of this book makes recommenda-tions for organizations that offer these materials.

Most important, emphasize that a dementia diagnosis doesn't mean someone has lost all skills, habits, pas-sions, likes, dislikes or the desire to be involved with life and connected with others. Let others know that the person with dementia can still do many or most things, sometimes with a little support or a few accommoda-tions. You may also explain that social interaction is necessary for the person's well-being; it's healthy for the brain, so it's important for the person living with dementia to stay engaged.

To meet practical needs, offer specific examples of ways people can help. The more specific you are about your needs, the better. For example, you might say, "We're looking for help getting to doctor appointments, and here are the scheduled times." If people ask how they can help, be prepared to answer.

You may want to post updates to keep people aware of your loved one's condition. Look to your local Alzheimer's Association chapter or a related organization for ideas regarding information that may be helpful to include in updates.

Finally, as you consider the needs of the person living with dementia, remember to keep your own needs in mind, as well. Friends who can provide conversation, emotional support and assistance can be invaluable.

2

Charting a path forward

When trying to navigate care for someone with dementia, care partners sometimes describe a strained, frustrating experience, including having trouble communicating with health care professionals. In part, this may be because the care partner isn't the patient, so privacy issues come into play.

At the same time, the person with dementia may not always provide the whole picture. For example, people with dementia may not accurately report the reality of their day-to-day experience or may lack good insight into their changes or needs. (See "What it means to have limited insight" on page 14.) In these situations, family care partners may not feel like they can disagree or contradict the person with dementia out of respect or because they don't want to cause an argument or distress. As a result, care partners may lose an opportunity to address their most pressing concerns.

As someone who's supporting a person living with dementia, you need to feel heard, validated and acknowledged — but you may need to overcome some obstacles to achieve this. Privacy regulations may limit the health care provider's ability to talk about a patient's condition with you unless appropriate authorizations are in place. Further, some health care providers may not want to talk about difficult topics, such as driving, because they're concerned it will impact their relationship with their patients. Or they may feel they don't have enough time or resources to fully address the care partner's questions or concerns.

Despite these realities, care partners can create a positive and productive health care experience with this advice.

FILL OUT THE PROPER PAPERWORK

Complete documents that allow health care professionals to talk with you about your loved one's care. These documents generally include a form that allows the release of medical information and a durable power of attorney (POA) for health care and medical decisions. These documents designate who can discuss diagnoses, treatments and other medical concerns.

A POA is a legal document that gives a person the power to make decisions for a person who's unable to do so. The person named in the POA may be a spouse, another family member, a friend or a member of a faith community. If you've been named in the POA, you can be involved in your loved one's treatment decisions. However, a POA doesn't mean that your loved one loses the ability to make decisions while still able to do so. As mental capacity decreases, a POA ensures that a person's best interests are honored. It may help to choose one or more alternates for a POA if the person named in this document becomes unable to fulfill the role.

PREPARE FOR APPOINTMENTS

Before each appointment, make a list of all over-the-counter drugs, prescription medications and supplements your loved one is taking each day, complete with doses. Bring a log of any changes, new symptoms or concerns you've witnessed. The log should include specific details, such as when you first noticed the change, when it happens or what triggers it.

Help make the best use of your time with your health care team by listing your specific concerns in the order of those you wish to discuss first. Listing your concerns in order of importance will help ensure that your most pressing needs are addressed.

Finally, bring a notepad to your appointment to take notes that you can refer to afterward.

MAKE SURE YOU AND YOUR LOVED ONE ARE HEARD

Don't be afraid to speak up, ask for what you want and share your point of view. As a care partner, you may not see yourself as an expert in dementia, but you *are* an expert in knowing the person you're supporting and what works best for him or her. As a care partner, your voice is critical. Health care professionals need your insight.

Help your loved one have a voice and feel heard and respected. We all want to be in charge of our own health and health care decisions; people living with dementia are no different. When attending an appointment, position yourself as your loved one's advocate and partner rather than the authority. Communicate in a way that sends a message that your loved one is respected and integral to the conversation and to the decisions that are made.

Here are some ways to do this:
- Include your loved one in the conversation. Don't speak as if your loved one isn't in the room; instead,

WHEN IT'S "SHOWTIME"

Sometimes, a person with dementia behaves or performs at a level significantly higher than their typical state for a short period of time. This is described as showtime. Showtime usually happens when people with dementia are with people who are outside their typical social circle, such as when they are visiting with a friend or distant relative ... or are in a doctor's office.

Showtime can be frustrating for you as a care partner when you need validation. When showtime happens, you may think the health care team feels that you're exaggerating the issues you're seeing or that you are the true problem.

Showtime mostly happens in the early stages of dementia and can happen for many reasons. Just being aware of showtime can help you cope with it. Consider keeping a journal of your day-to-day observations. This can help you capture specific details to discuss with your health care team.

ask for your loved one's thoughts and opinions. You may need to do some on-the-spot education with the doctor if your loved one talks only to you.

- Don't interrupt. People with dementia may need extra time to express what they want to say.
- Adopt the mindset that no matter what happens, you will avoid confronting or arguing. Arguing with a person who has dementia rarely, if ever, results in a good outcome.

CREATE A PLAN TO STAY IN TOUCH

It's not always practical to make an appointment or wait until an office visit to talk about issues, ask questions or share information. Ask your loved one's health care team about how to stay in touch between visits. You may rely on a nurse, social worker, care navigator or another member of the health care team to serve as your point of contact. You may set up a phone call with the doctor ahead of an appointment. Or an email or online service like a secure website or patient portal may be an option.

If you have information to share privately and haven't been able to get in touch with your loved one's health care team before an appointment, consider writing a note and giving it to a nurse or another staff person when you get to the appointment and asking that the doctor read the note before entering the exam room.

LET THE DOCTOR TAKE THE BLAME

If your loved one doesn't think it's necessary to stop driving or take a certain medication or do something else that's important for health and well-being, let it be the doctor's directive. As a care partner, you need to preserve your relationship with your loved one. In these instances, you aren't agreeing with your loved one. Instead, you're validating how the person with dementia feels about it. It's always better to listen, validate and respond with empathy — all things you'll learn more about as you continue to read this book. You may say something like, "The doctor said you need to stop driving. I'm sorry this is making you feel so angry. This must be hard."

CONNECT WITH YOUR OWN HEALTH CARE PROVIDER

It's important that you have your own health care provider and maintain regular visits to meet your health care needs. During these visits, be honest about what you're going through as a caregiver and any feelings you have, such as sadness, worry or anxiety. Your health care provider may be able to recommend virtual and in-person support groups for care partners who support people living with dementia. These sources of support can be an effective way to reduce your feelings of isolation as well as learn from others in a caregiving role. Later in this book, you'll learn about other ways to get the support you need.

PLANNING FOR THE FUTURE

Coming to terms with a dementia diagnosis takes time. Later in this book, you'll learn ways to adjust to the care partner role. Once the reality of the situation sinks in a little and you're ready to do so, give some thought to the future. Making preparations early on allows you to create carefully considered plans that address your loved one's changing needs. It also gives the person with dementia the best opportunity to make shared decisions with you and other family members. Here are several steps to take.

Get affairs in order

Whether you have dementia or not, it's a good idea to complete important legal documents that allow you to communicate your wishes about the kind of medical care and treatment you want to receive. These documents also designate someone to make medical decisions on an individual's behalf when the individual is unable to do so. You'll get tips for completing these documents in Chapter 9.

Make a financial plan

The costs of immediate and long-term dementia care can be daunting. These costs may include treatment for dementia and other medical conditions, medications, in-home services, adult day care, and skilled residential care in settings such as memory care communities or nursing homes. While medical and other insurance may help to defray health care costs, many don't cover expenses for services such as home-based care, adult day care and assisted living.

Addressing your financial future sooner than later helps reduce stress. The following steps can help you plan ahead for the costs of dementia care.

Get the lay of the land

Personal savings, investments and property can be sources of income to help pay for dementia care now and in the future. To start, review all financial and legal documents, including:

- Living wills.
- Wills.
- Medical and durable powers of attorney, including mental health power of attorney.
- Bank and brokerage accounts.
- Deeds, mortgage papers or ownership statements.
- Pension and other retirement benefit summaries.
- Social Security payment information.
- Stock and bond certificates.
- Monthly or outstanding bills.
- Insurance policies.

Going over these documents can help you understand your current expenses, income and assets, as well as how future financial and medical decisions will be handled. A document review can also reveal any important legal documents, such as a living will or powers of attorney, that may still need to be put in place.

If you have a workplace flexible spending account (FSA) and your loved one is a dependent under tax rules, you may be able to use the FSA to cover your loved one's medical costs or dependent care expenses. Contact your FSA plan's customer service department to ask about this option.

Investigate additional sources of financial support

You may be able to cover some medical and care costs if your loved one qualifies for federal and state government assistance, such as:

- Social Security Administration programs, including Social Security Disability Income (SSDI) and Supplemental Security Income (SSI).

- Health care benefits from the Department of Veterans Affairs.
- Medicare or Medicaid.
- Program of All-Inclusive Care for the Elderly (PACE), a Medicare program.

Find contact information for these organizations in the Resources section of this book.

The National Council on Aging offers a free benefits checkup service that can help you find federal and state benefit programs you may be eligible for. Visit www.benefitscheckup.org to learn more. If you use Medicare or Medicaid, the national State Health Insurance Assistance Program (SHIP) can also provide guidance on these benefits.

Community-based organizations may be another source of support. Some local nonprofits offer free or low-cost services, such as meal delivery, rides to medical appointments and respite care.

Get advice from a professional

Consider consulting with a financial planner, an attorney who specializes in estates or an accountant who is knowledgeable about payment plans for care alternatives. It may be helpful to work with someone who also specializes in elder care or terminal illness issues. These professionals can help determine if you're eligible for tax deductions and financial resources. A professional may also help you avoid bad investment decisions that could deplete your finances.

When choosing a financial adviser, be sure to check qualifications, such as professional credentials, education and membership in professional associations. For help finding an adviser, try these resources:

- The Eldercare Locator.
- The Alzheimer's Association & AARP Community Resource Finder.
- The Financial Planning Association's PlannerSearch directory.
- The Certified Financial Planner Board of Standards.
- The National Academy of Elder Law Attorneys.

Learn more in the Resources section of this book.

Think long-term

Many care partners wonder what they'll do if their loved one's disease becomes severe enough that caregiving in the home is no longer feasible. Rather than wait until that time comes, plan ahead. Early planning gives you time to study the resources in your community. It may also enable you to ask the person with dementia about personal preferences for future care.

Just as important, planning ahead allows you to learn about the costs of long-term care outside the home. Some costs may be covered if your loved one enrolled in long-term care insurance before receiving a dementia diagnosis. In many cases, though, skilled care in a long-term care community is an out-of-pocket expense. Knowing the costs up front can help you make decisions and create a realistic financial plan.

Plan for emergencies

Sometimes the unexpected happens. You get injured or sick, or an accident temporarily disrupts your life and your ability to support the person in your care. Planning ahead for this type of emergency can reduce stress for both you and your loved one.

Talk to trusted friends, neighbors or family members. They may be happy to serve as backup caregivers in an emergency. Respite care services can be another option. Respite care comes in several forms.

In-home care

In-home respite care providers may offer companionship and supervision, assistance with daily grooming or skilled care for certain medical needs.

Adult day centers

Adult day centers provide supervised activities outside the home for a few hours a day, for as many days as you choose. Some centers are designed specifically for people living with dementia.

Residential respite

Certain skilled-care residential communities may provide overnight respite care for several days or even a few weeks.

It can be challenging to identify the various sources of respite care in your area, especially if you're trying to find support on short notice. Learning in advance about agencies that provide respite services on an emergency basis will help you in the event that you need to call on them. (See "Finding support services" on page 41 for tips on how to start your search.) Once you've located providers that offer emergency care, consider register-

FINDING SUPPORT SERVICES

Support services in your area can be invaluable. These types of services include daily or longer-term care, respite services, transportation and meal delivery and support groups.

Your loved one's health care team may be able to recommend local service providers and support groups. You may also want to enlist the help of a professional, such as a geriatric case manager. A geriatric case manager is usually a nurse or social worker who can recommend or help coordinate care services. Some local government agencies and charities offer geriatric care consulting services for free or for a sliding-scale fee.

In addition, these organizations help families identify local dementia and elder care resources:
• Dementia advocacy organizations such as the Alzheimer's Association and the Alzheimer's Foundation of America.
• The Eldercare Locator, a public service offered by the U.S. Administration on Aging.
• Nonprofits such as the National Adult Day Services Association and the ARCH National Respite Network.

Find more information on these organizations in the Resources section of this book.

ing with one or more of them. You may even want to try out these providers in nonemergency situations to see how well their services work. Occasionally using a respite care provider can also help a person with dementia become more comfortable with the experience.

Recharge with respite care

Keep in mind that respite care can also support care partners in everyday life. Using a service for planned breaks allows you to recharge in whatever way helps you most. The person with dementia may also benefit from the additional companionship and enjoyable activities that respite care provides.

MANY WAYS TO MOVE FORWARD

Adjusting to a diagnosis and planning for the future are key steps to adapting to life with Alzheimer's disease and other forms of dementia. Another vital step is to find ways to optimize well-being. Well-being is critical for people living with dementia, as well as their care partners. The next few chapters offer valuable information and strategies.

3

What it means to be a caregiver

When Nick was diagnosed with Alzheimer's disease, the doctor turned to his wife, Marie, and referred to her as his caregiver. Marie was rattled. "I'm Nick's wife," she said. "When did that change?"

When does the label *caregiver* replace *wife*? If your husband or wife is diagnosed with dementia, do you leave the doctor's office with a new label, title and role? When do spouses label themselves as caregivers?

To a large degree, people rely on labels to define themselves. Labels connect people to their identities and self-worth: wife, husband, father, daughter, artist, vegetarian.

Often, these labels don't necessarily reflect who people are as much as what they do, their social status or how they function in life. In a society that puts so much emphasis on the desire to be something, each person grapples with figuring out exactly who they are in relation to the world. Even more important, the language or words people use to describe themselves influence their thoughts, their emotions, their expectations and their behaviors.

In Marie's case, instead of *being* a caregiver, she may choose to see herself as a wife in a caring or supportive role — a care partner or support partner. Like Marie, most people don't want caregiving to define who they are. However, identifying as a caregiver or a care partner may actually be a good thing.

By identifying yourself in this way, you start to pay attention to information, resources and services that can help you. Most important, you become part of a larger group of people with common issues, needs and concerns. You begin to build recognition not of who you are but of what you do. When you can name and label one of your roles, you can validate your experiences and nurture your feelings.

By calling yourself a care partner, you're saying to the world, "Here I am. Acknowledge me, hear me, support me. I matter."

CHALLENGES AND BENEFITS OF CAREGIVING

Most people who care for those living with dementia are spouses, adult children and other relatives and friends. These people are referred to as informal or family caregivers.

Across the United States, family members, friends and other unpaid care partners are contributing billions of hours to the care of loved ones living with Alzheimer's disease or other dementias.

Among these care partners, approximately two-thirds are women, and about a third are 65 or older. Around half of all care partners are caring for a parent. About 1 in 4 belongs to the sandwich genera-

CAREGIVER OR CARE PARTNER?

The term *care partner* acknowledges the reciprocal relationship that can continue to exist between a person with dementia and a spouse, partner or other relative.

Learning to approach support and caring as a partnership means seeing the person with dementia as a whole human being and not making assumptions based on a diagnosis or label. It means including the person with dementia in decision-making. It also means making adaptations so people living with dementia can continue to live life to the best of their abilities.

The term *caregiver* better describes a role in which the caring responsibility moves to a place beyond partnering and includes more care *giving*. The person with dementia is just as much of an individual as before but has become more dependent on the care of another.

tion. People in this group are caring for both an older adult and children under 18.

Care partners provide support in a variety of ways. They may help with activities of daily living, from household chores, meal preparation and transportation to bathing, dressing and grooming. They may need to help ensure that medications are being taken correctly and other treatment regimens are being followed. They provide emotional support and may need to address changing behaviors like confusion and nighttime disturbances. Care partners may also hire and oversee paid care for their loved ones in the home or in other care communities.

These supportive tasks can take a toll on a care partner, especially as the disease progresses. Compared with those who care for people living with other conditions and illnesses, dementia care partners may be more likely to experience emotional stress, anxiety and depression. This is particularly true when the person living with dementia is a spouse.

Because caring for someone with dementia can lead to chronic stress, care partners may experience a variety of health problems. Poor sleep, a weaker immune system, high blood pressure (hypertension) and heart disease are examples. Care partners may also be more at risk of developing cognitive issues, including memory decline. On the other hand, many people caring for someone with dementia say that their own health is excellent or very good.

Despite its challenges, being a care partner may have some positive effects. Playing such a vital role in a loved one's life can be deeply gratifying. Many care partners feel a sense of accomplishment and purpose and say that they have experienced positive personal growth. In two recent surveys, most care partners said that although caring for someone with

CAREGIVER'S BILL OF RIGHTS

Being a care partner comes with its share of ups and downs. It's easy to lose yourself in the needs of your loved one, pushing your own needs, feelings and desires aside. But you can't be an effective care partner if you're always putting yourself last.

Advocates for caregivers and the people they care for have developed a set of rights they believe caregivers are entitled to. These include the right to:
- Maintain your sense of self as an individual by leading your life with dignity.
- Know self-care is not selfishness and it's important to nurture a life outside your care partner role.
- Make decisions about your loved one that reflect the needs and promote the well-being of you both.
- Be recognized for the vital role you play in your family and in your loved one's life.
- Treat yourself with love and compassion so that you can reject guilt or doubt and be confident that you're caring for your loved one to the best of your abilities.

Alzheimer's disease or other dementias is demanding, it's also rewarding, fulfilling and meaningful. Some care partners also say that the experience has brought them closer to the person living with dementia and to other family members.

THE TERM *LOVED ONE* DOESN'T ALWAYS FIT

Care partners experience their roles in different ways depending on many factors involved in their relationship with someone living with dementia. Caring for a spouse with whom you have a loving relationship is one example of a care partner relationship. For this reason, in this book you'll notice that people living with dementia are sometimes referred to as loved ones. In many cases, the person with dementia that you're caring for is, indeed, someone you love.

In other cases, however, the term *loved one* doesn't quite fit a care partner's unique situation. There are many other types of relationships that care partners find themselves in. For example, you may be providing care and support to someone you've had an estranged or troubled relationship with.

For this reason, the terms *loved one* and *person living with dementia* are used interchangeably in this book to represent the breadth of relationships that care partners have with those living with dementia.

AN UNREQUESTED ROLE

When a parent or spouse develops dementia, it naturally begins to change the dynamics of your relationship. You may feel scared, uncertain or even resentful. You may feel as if you've been plunged into a role you never asked for and don't feel prepared to take on. Your loved one with dementia is also likely dealing with this shift in roles and the impact it might have on the relationship.

Adapting to the role of care partner has many dimensions, depending on how your relationship has functioned in the past. In time, you may need to assume responsibilities your loved one has taken pride in handling. For example, you may need to start paying the bills, mowing the lawn or shopping for groceries. If those tasks weren't your responsibility before, this can be a challenge.

You may also become responsible for matters that your loved one considers personal and private. Adult children, in particular, often hesitate to make decisions for parents, including moving them from a private home to an assisted living community.

Taking on this new role as a care partner doesn't mean the end of a relationship, only that the relationship will change, as all relationships do over time. Adapting to these changes involves emotional adjustments. Take heart in knowing that others have walked in your shoes and experienced similar feelings. Find hope in knowing that some care partners have not only adapted to their roles as care partners but also discovered an inner strength, patience and resiliency they didn't know they had.

What if the past relationship between a care partner and the person with dementia has been rocky? Certainly, previous differences will impact how you think about the care partner role now.

Although it's never easy, it's important to let go of the past and those feelings and thoughts that no longer serve you. They will only sap your energy and weigh you down. When you make the choice to let go

EXPRESSING AFFECTION AND INTIMACY WITH YOUR SPOUSE OR PARTNER

Expressions of affection, whether sexual or nonsexual, are essential for the well-being of both you and your loved one. The need for closeness doesn't lessen with age or with cognitive decline. Yet like any relationship, the connection you share with your spouse or partner is complex and ever-changing.

You may notice that the effects of the disease or its treatment cause your loved one to experience an increase or decrease in sex drive. At the same time, you may feel a range of emotions about sexual intimacy in your relationship.

If your loved one shows less interest in sex, you might feel rejected or lonely. In contrast, you may feel guilty if your desire to interact sexually with your loved one wanes as the disease progresses. It's common for a caregiver to lose sexual desire for a spouse who has dementia for many reasons, of a negative past and work toward accepting the way life is today, things can improve.

Your new role in supporting a person living with dementia can give you the chance to create a new — and sometimes even improved — relationship.

including the demands of the caregiver role and the transition from intimate partner to caregiver.

Caregivers should not feel guilty if their sexual desire has changed.

If you're experiencing difficult or conflicting feelings, it can help to talk about them with your spouse or partner. Build a new relationship slowly, and use your instincts to determine whether the experience is pleasurable for both of you. If you still have concerns, consider talking to a mental health provider.

Regardless of your situation, touch is a powerful tool that you can use to maintain an important sense of closeness and connection. Touch can be experienced in many ways, including holding hands and hugging.

4

Overcoming common caregiver challenges

I struggle to adjust and adapt to so many changes. I feel so angry. Frustrated. Everything is such an endeavor. Explaining, reexplaining and then going over it all again. I keep reminding myself to go slow, stay calm and take it easy. I am not doing so great in this role. I want to run away. I feel like I am in quicksand and can't find solid ground.

This reflection comes from Rosalie, a care partner to her husband, who has Lewy body dementia — but it could be the experience of many caregivers. The role of a care partner can be emotionally and physically exhausting. There may be many moments of frustration, anxiety and tension for everyone involved.

It's essential to keep in mind that, like you, a person with dementia is a whole, multifaceted person doing the best in the face of challenges. There are many things you can do as a care partner to help the person you're supporting live the best life possible with dementia. This chapter offers practical advice for addressing challenging situations and overcoming obstacles. You'll also learn how to employ a whole-person approach to your life, which offers benefits for you as well as the person living with dementia.

LEARN EVERYTHING YOU CAN

The more you understand about dementia, the more able you'll be to make a positive impact. Disease-related changes will seem less mysterious, and you may find it easier to adapt caregiving responsibilities so that your days feel more manageable. Knowing more about dementia can also help you feel confident in making important decisions about how to live your life and plan for the future.

At the same time, it's critical to think beyond the disease itself and focus on the whole person, an approach sometimes defined as person-centered care.

Social psychologist Thomas Kitwood first used the term *person-centered care* in the late 1980s to define a philosophy of care that's different from standard medical and behavioral care.

Today, many experts prefer the terms *individualized care* and *personalized care*, but the idea is the same: a focus on the whole person. This means not just focusing on the disease or the diagnosis but also seeking to know and appreciate a person's past and present roles in life, preferences, beliefs, values and needs. A person-centered approach offers a balanced perspective that can help with many of the challenges of dementia.

Relationships are especially important in person-centered care. All human beings are born to relate, connect and bond, and these needs remain for a lifetime. Having dementia doesn't change this, but dementia does make it more difficult to sustain quality relationships and meaningful engagement.

FOCUS ON WELL-BEING

Quality of life is related to a person's overall well-being. Researchers have described well-being for people with dementia in terms of comfort, inclusion, identity, occupation and attachment. More recently, Alzheimer's Disease International defined *well-being* as feeling content, being happy, feeling safe, experiencing pleasure and joy, and having a sense of self-worth and purpose. The opposite of well-being, in contrast, is described as suffering, pain, distress, fear, loneliness and humiliation.

To support the growing body of research on this topic, G. Allen Power, M.D., an international expert in models of care for older adults living with dementia, translates well-being into seven domains: identity, connectedness, security, autonomy, meaning, growth and joy.

No matter how you define *well-being*, focusing on it may contribute more to quality of life for people living with dementia than any medication available today. Despite their disease, people with dementia can experience well-being, and they can continue to grow and learn. Well-being is within reach when care partners, families and communities all play an active role.

As dementia progresses, daily tasks such as dressing, bathing and mealtimes can become more difficult.

Having a plan with practical strategies to get through the day can help. Take the values and preferences of the person living with dementia into consideration, along with the following suggestions. Remember that each person living with dementia is unique and will respond differently, so it may take time and a bit of trial and error. Also, what works now may change as the disease changes.

OFFER EMPATHY

To empathize means to imagine, as best as you can, what it's like to live someone else's life and to seek to understand another person's experience and reality.

Showing empathy can improve life for someone living with dementia, and it's good for a care partner's well-being too. Research suggests that when people caring for someone with dementia use empathy, they're less likely to feel depressed. One of the most important things you can do as a care partner is to seek to understand your loved one's experience and reality.

Reality can be distorted for people living with dementia; trying to make them fit within your reality will cause stress for everyone involved. This doesn't mean that people living with dementia are far away or lost, but it does mean that the disease impacts the ability of a person with dementia to communicate clearly and process the world in the same way you do.

Seeing life through the eyes of the person with dementia doesn't mean you have to share the same anxiety, sadness or agitation. It also doesn't mean you have to lie or agree with the person's sense of reality (see page 72). Healthy empathy involves listening and observing with your ears, eyes and heart and means accepting that your reality may be different.

Genuine empathy is expressed in your tone of voice, your eyes and your curiosity toward understanding your loved one's world from their view of reality. Empathy is offered in your silence, your observing and your listening. Showing empathy helps others feel that there is a space for them just as they are.

RECOGNIZE STRENGTHS AND POTENTIAL

Every person living with dementia will experience dementia in a different way. Part of this experience includes retaining certain strengths and abilities. It's a myth that a diagnosis of dementia automatically means people can't do any of the things they used to do or can't learn new things.

People living with dementia have preserved abilities and areas of strength despite their disease. To truly help a person with dementia, it's important to focus on the person's best qualities, rather than only on what the person has lost or can no longer do. Although each type of dementia has a typical pattern of progression, people experience dementia differently. An individual's experiences, skills and interests all contribute to preserved strengths. Even late in the disease, people with dementia can maintain and express a full range of emotions, including pleasure, enjoyment and affection. They often have a sense of humor they can still tap into.

Recognizing and building on strengths and abilities is an important way to nurture well-being in people living with dementia. Following are a few key areas of strength.

Strength: Procedural memory

The ability to store and recall memories is affected in many types of dementia. Take Alzheimer's dementia, for example. It affects the ability to form memories of new knowledge and events. Recalling a conversation from earlier in the day or remembering what you ate for dinner last night could be a challenge with Alzheimer's. This could cause the person with dementia to feel embarrassed or frustrated.

But people with Alzheimer's dementia can make and recall new memories by using procedural memory. Procedural memory is a type of long-term memory that allows someone to perform different actions and use certain skills. It's created by repeating an activity or skill until it becomes automatic and doesn't require conscious thought. Tying your shoes, riding a bike and brushing your teeth are examples of procedural memory.

In Alzheimer's dementia, procedural memory is more resilient than other types of memory. Some people with dementia can maintain procedural memories for quite some time and learn new things by tapping into the way these memories are formed.

Accountants and math teachers, for example, may retain their numbers skills longer than other people with dementia because they represent an overlearned skill — something they did daily almost without thinking. Likewise, people who played golf or bowled for decades may be able to play the game well into their disease. Overlearned skills tend to remain intact even as a person progresses into the middle and sometimes later stages of dementia. Other examples of overlearned tasks include making a bed, riding a bike, caring for an animal and folding laundry. Every individual has a set of procedural skills.

Strength: Emotional memory

Everyone feels emotions, even without recalling what sparked them. The ability to experience and maintain emotions, as well as to accurately perceive others'

ELEANOR'S STORY: USING PROCEDURAL MEMORY TO LEARN SOMETHING NEW

Eleanor was living with Alzheimer's dementia. She and her family decided she would move from the assisted living community where she'd been for two years to a different care community a few miles away. The move went as smoothly as could be expected, and Eleanor settled into her new home. She was a bit apprehensive, but still eager to be involved in all the activities this community had to offer.

But there was a problem. Eleanor lived on the third floor, and most of the daily activities and opportunities for socializing happened on the first floor. When Eleanor left her apartment in search of something to do, she got lost. When she couldn't find her way downstairs, she became frustrated and angry. When she was offered assistance, she said she didn't need anyone's help.

After a couple of days, staff members came up with a plan. They applied large adhesive footprint decals on the floor leading from Eleanor's apartment door to the elevator. Inside the elevator, they placed a sign next to the first-floor button that read, "Activity room, press here." At the elevator opening on the first floor, more footprint decals were placed, leading to the emotions, remains intact for many people with dementia throughout the stages of their disease. This is particularly true for people living with Alzheimer's dementia. With the right communication, you can create a meaningful visit that leaves a positive, lasting emotional

activity room. Eleanor was able to successfully follow the footprints to and from her apartment every day, sometimes several times a day.

The fact that Eleanor could find her way by using these simple visual cues may not come as a surprise, but what happened next might. After about six weeks, the staff removed the footprint decals and waited to see what would happen. At her usual time, without any sign of frustration, Eleanor arrived in the activity room like she had every day for the past six weeks.

Eleanor was able to find her way, without the assistance of the footprint decals, by using procedural memory. Repeatedly and successfully going back and forth between her apartment and the activity room for six weeks helped Eleanor learn this route, which essentially imprinted a new memory in her brain.

Eleanor's story highlights the overall benefits of repetition and establishing a daily routine. These habits support new learning and can help someone with dementia remain more independent and feel less frustrated and anxious.

impact. (Learn more about communication skills starting on page 68.)

That being said, emotional memory also includes bad memories. If you say or do something that causes emotional distress for a person with dementia, those

EMOTIONS LAST LONG AFTER MEMORIES FADE

In a study from the University of Iowa, researchers asked individuals living with Alzheimer's dementia to watch film clips that were intended to make them feel either sad or happy. The researchers collected emotion ratings at three different points, and after each point, they gave a memory test. Participants had trouble recalling details about the film clips; some couldn't remember a single detail about the film. However, feelings of happiness and sadness evoked by the film were remembered.

This study is consistent with other research suggesting that people living with significant memory issues can be emotionally affected by an event even if they can't recall the event itself. These emotions can last long after memories have faded.

This offers an important lesson for care partners, friends and community members alike. People living with dementia may not remember your name, recognize your face or recall how they know you, but that doesn't change how much your visits and interactions matter.

emotions can persist long after the situation that triggered the distress is forgotten. This may explain why certain people or places cause a negative reaction in someone with dementia. The person may be responding to something that happened days, weeks or even months ago.

If you think it won't be worthwhile to visit a person with dementia simply because the person won't remember it, think again. People with dementia live in the moment and will enjoy the time you spend together. Your visit can generate positive feelings that may linger well past your time together.

Strength: Art and creativity

"The arts are a way of being in relationship that can ensure that we are more than our diagnosis," says Anne Basting, Ph.D., a scholar, author and artist. Her work focuses on how the arts can transform the lives of those living with dementia. Her words describe the impact that the arts can make on people with dementia.

More and more evidence points to the benefits the arts have for those living with dementia. Whether it's visual art, music, dance, storytelling, poetry or anything else that evokes creativity and imagination, the arts can reduce stress and improve quality of life for those living with dementia and for their care partners.

There are many reasons for this. For one, intuition, creativity and imagination are areas of strength for people with dementia. The ability to appreciate, produce and participate in art isn't affected by their disease. And because most art doesn't require specific memories or traditional language use, it allows people with dementia to express feelings they may not be able to communicate verbally.

Research shows that in people living with dementia, art therapy can engage attention, bring a sense of pleasure, improve symptoms like agitation, aggression, depression and apathy and improve self-esteem and social behavior.

Creativity can even emerge in people with dementia. In fact, depending on how and where dementia affects the brain, artistic ability may even be enhanced in people with a certain type of frontotemporal dementia as the disease progresses.

Music is another example of how the arts can benefit people living with dementia. Despite profound memory loss, individuals with dementia often show a remarkable memory for music. That's because the areas of the brain that process and remember music are typically less damaged by dementia than other regions. Music also tends to arouse emotions and influence mood. For many, music retains this power throughout the disease.

Research suggests that listening to or singing songs can offer benefits for people with dementia. Music can relieve stress, reduce anxiety and depression and lessen agitation. Certain types of music can be calming, while other types can help boost mood.

Worldwide, organizations like the Giving Voice Initiative use music to bring people living with Alzheimer's and their care partners together to sing in choruses that foster joy, well-being, purpose and community understanding. Find groups dedicated to the arts listed in the Resources section of this book.

UNDERSTAND AND REDUCE DISTRESS

Human beings all need to feel respected, worthy and connected. Although these emotional needs are universal, people with dementia struggle to have these needs met.

Imagine what it would feel like to wake up one day and discover that you could no longer take part in the things that give your life meaning and purpose. Or think about how you'd feel if people suddenly started telling you what you could and couldn't do. How would you feel if you could no longer make basic choices for yourself, like choosing when to have your morning cup of coffee or with whom you share a meal?

These are examples of the reality that many people with dementia face — a reality that understandably leads to feelings of apathy, anger and frustration.

Imagine the following:
- Having someone you don't know show up and tell you that they will be giving you a bath.
- Feeling bored and no longer able to do the things that give you a sense of worth or purpose.
- Someone with a grimacing face talking at you in a patronizing tone, in a language you can't understand.
- Being uncomfortable or in pain, or needing to find the bathroom, and being unable to find the words to ask for help.
- Feeling tired and wanting to find your way home so you can rest. Instead, you're stuck in a confusing, cluttered space with chatter, sounds and dozens of people you don't recognize.
- Being treated as if you can't do something that, with a little more time and patience, you could probably do just fine.

Thinking about what it might feel like to be in these situations can help you empathize with a person living with dementia. Would you feel agitated, angry, anxious, scared, hopeless or sad? If you said yes, know that someone with dementia feels this way too.

EMOTIONAL WELL-BEING CHECKLIST

Like all people, people living with dementia have the need to:

- **Feel respected.** Always treat someone with dementia as an adult, under all circumstances. This includes your actions, as well as your verbal and nonverbal communication.
- **Feel needed and have purpose.** Find ways to help people with dementia feel valued and productive by helping them to engage in things that have meaning to them. Ask for their help, advice and opinions daily.
- **Feel connected and have a sense of belonging.** Recognize the importance of having strong, supportive relationships. Play a role in helping the person living with dementia maintain friendships or find new opportunities for support and belonging.
- **Feel good about themselves.** Offer honest appreciation and praise every day for traits and accomplishments large or small.
- **Have choice and control.** Involve the person with dementia in decisions every day. Think about doing things *with* rather than always doing things *for* the person with dementia. Ask the person with dementia for permission.

Many dementia advocates are working to improve social and emotional health for people living with dementia. You can help in your own way. Use the checklist on the previous page to gauge how well you're helping fulfill the emotional needs of someone living with dementia. The next time you notice anger, agitation, apathy, frustration or any type of distress, this list may provide clues as to the cause.

Decoding distress

Many people find changes in behavior to be the most challenging aspect of dementia. Depression, apathy, anxiety, agitation, aggression, sleep disturbances and poorly controlled emotions or actions are all examples. Anywhere from a third to nearly all people with dementia will experience some or many of these symptoms.

What causes these behaviors — and how to address them — isn't always clear. But part of the answer lies in understanding the changes in the brain. Certain brain circuits have been linked to a tendency toward certain symptoms, like apathy, delusions and agitation. Not everyone with dementia will develop these symptoms; this continues to be an area of study for researchers.

Over time, dementia changes how well people can communicate their needs and provide for themselves. Behaviors become a way to communicate. Anger or agitation, for example, are expressions of distress and can be a way for people living with dementia to say they're in pain or feeling misunderstood, confused, disrespected or bored.

For understanding the exact cause of distress in someone with dementia, empathy becomes essential.

COMMON CAUSES OF DISTRESS

Use these checklists to spot common causes of distress for people living with dementia.

Physical needs
A common physical problem is pain. Others include needing to go to the bathroom, not seeing or hearing well, and feeling uncomfortable or too hot or too cold. A person with dementia may communicate physical discomfort through behaviors or expressions rather than with words.

Nonverbal signs of pain may include the following:
- Grimacing.
- Gestures.
- Moaning.
- Restlessness.
- Crying.
- Expressions of distress, like agitation or aggression.

The environment
While a person's environment can promote comfort, independence and overall well-being, it can also increase agitation and other reactions.

Environmental factors that can cause distress include the following:
- Feeling too hot or too cold.
- Lack of structure or routine.
- Too much noise or overstimulation.
- Too much clutter.

- Too much quiet.
- New or confusing surroundings.
- Poor lighting.

Emotional needs

A person with dementia may be feeling bored, unworthy or disconnected from the people and things that provide purpose. When these needs aren't met, overall well-being and quality of life decrease.

Signs of emotional distress may include expressions like agitation or apathy.

Communication challenges

Changes in the brain caused by dementia make communication more difficult over time. In moderate stages of dementia, it can be increasingly difficult to understand what someone with dementia is saying. In this chapter, you'll learn ways to improve your communication skills.

You may notice changes like these:
- Trouble finding the right word and leaving thoughts hanging in midsentence.
- Words, sentences and thoughts become jumbled.
- What you say isn't easily understood, leading to embarrassment, anger or agitation.
- Verbal communication may be replaced by nonverbal communication, including behaviors, sounds, facial expressions and gestures.

Empathy, as you learned earlier, is the ability to imagine, as best you can, what it's like to live with dementia. This includes how someone with dementia may be perceiving the world in that moment.

Decoding distress means operating from the belief that most behavior is reasonable based on the circumstances. There's meaning behind it, and it's often triggered by something or someone. Start by asking yourself, *I wonder what could be causing this distress?* Instead of assuming that a behavior is an expected symptom of dementia, think of the behavior as an attempt to express distress or communicate an unmet need. You may feel like a detective looking for clues, but with a little effort, you can often uncover the cause. Once you can identify the likely cause, solutions become possible.

COMMUNICATE SKILLFULLY

Although ways of communicating will change as dementia progresses, you can develop new and effective ways to communicate with your loved one. Along the way, you may even learn some things about yourself and strengthen qualities like patience and acceptance. Effective communication is essential to everyone's well-being.

Start with these basic strategies for good communication.
- Talk to a person with dementia as an adult, in an adult tone of voice and with words that are respectful.
- Face the person before you communicate. Look directly at the person and make eye contact.
- Speak at your usual volume or a little louder if listening conditions are difficult.
- Slow the pace of your conversation. It takes more time for people with dementia to process information.
- Use words that are familiar and easy to picture in

your mind (concrete) rather than abstract words. Be clear and concise; keep your message short.

- Pause after a statement or question. Allow plenty of time for a response.
- Avoid leading questions that include the answer with it. "You're comfortable, aren't you?" is an example. This kind of question can be demeaning, and in some cases, the person will agree with anything you say.
- Use nonverbal cues, like smiling or giving a reassuring touch.
- Give instructions one step at a time. After one step is completed, give instructions for the next step.
- Don't interrupt. People with dementia may need extra time to express what they want to say. If the person is struggling to express a thought, gently offer a word or phrase.
- Take note of facial expressions and hand gestures. They may offer clues to forgotten words.
- Use gestures and show the object you're talking about if your words don't seem to be understood.
- Avoid criticizing, confronting or arguing. People with dementia experience the world in a different way, so it's unlikely that they'll see things the way you do all the time.
- Do not speak in the presence of a person with dementia as if the person is not there.

Aside from basic communication strategies, here are ways to communicate with someone living with dementia that tap into abilities that aren't affected by the disease.

Consider nonverbal cues

How you present yourself is critical. Are you nervous or frowning? Are you speaking clearly and simply? Is your facial expression or body language sending a negative message? The words you use are only part of the message you communicate.

Body language, facial expressions, posture, gestures and tone of voice are also factors that affect how your message is received. People living with dementia understand nonverbal communication well. Body language is an especially powerful way to send a message to someone with dementia.

Offer choice and sense of control

A sense of control is important for everyone. Yet people with dementia often feel as if they're being told what to do or that they're not capable of making their own decisions. This is another area where effective communication can make a difference.

Consider the following examples:

A. It's time for you to take your medication.
B. Would you like me to get you a glass of water so you can take your medication?

A. I need you to stay here while I get the car.
B. Would you like to stand here or sit in that chair while I get the car?

A. Let's go to the bathroom, Dad.
B. Dad, may I help you get to the bathroom?

A. No, that's not how you do it.
B. Here's another way.

Each of the A statements competes with a person's need for choice and control. When they're heard over and over again, these statements can cause someone with dementia to lose self-confidence and feel angry, agitated and even hopeless.

The B statements, on the other hand, offer choice, consider a person's preferences and preserve a person's need to feel respected.

Ask the right questions

As memory loss becomes more noticeable, avoid asking questions that depend on memory or that have only one right answer. Avoid saying, "Do you remember ... ?" Instead, ask questions that tap into your loved one's strengths.

Asking questions about a person's ideas, thoughts, feelings and preferences allows you to take full advantage of the areas of the brain that are less affected. It's important to keep in mind that not everyone will need the same adaptations in communication.

Here are examples of questions you might ask.

A. Do you remember what I told you to do today?
B. You agreed to rake the leaves this afternoon. Can I grab a rake for you?

A. This is a big menu. What do you want?
B. Both the fish special and the meatloaf look good tonight. What do you think?

A. How many grandchildren do you have?
B. How do you feel about having 14 grandchildren?

In these examples, the A statements rely on memory or require abstract thinking. The B statements, on the other hand, eliminate the need for remembering. They also offer clarity, give limited choices and ask about preferences.

Ask "beautiful" questions

Asking questions that depend on memory can cause feelings of shame and embarrassment for someone with dementia. That's where taking a different approach to the questions you ask — one that taps into the freedom of imagination — can be valuable.

• What is the greatest gift you could receive?
• What is the most beautiful sound in your home?

TO LIE OR NOT TO LIE

When someone with dementia believes something that's false, it can be hard to know what to say.

For example, let's say your mother has dementia and repeatedly asks where her husband is. The truth is that he died a year ago. Do you repeatedly tell her the truth, knowing that her reaction is going to be shock, grief and fear every time? Each time, it will be as if she's learning this news for the first time. Which is worse: telling a lie or offering the painful truth?

This is where an approach commonly called *therapeutic fibbing* may come into play. While this can be an effective strategy, it's also controversial. It means going along with or not correcting a misconception. The idea is to decrease worry, sadness, agitation or anxiety in someone with dementia.

- How would you welcome a new friend to your home?
- How does painting make you feel?
- What do you wish for?
- What are you thankful for?

These are all examples of "beautiful questions," a creative way of using arts and imagination to ask questions that engage people with dementia.

This concept comes from Anne Basting, Ph.D., founder and president of the nonprofit TimeSlips (www. timeslips.org). The TimeSlips website offers hundreds of prompts to inspire creative engagement. Basting also

For the situation described here, therapeutic fibbing may involve a response like, "When the weather is nice like today, your husband sometimes stays out in the fields after dark." This statement isn't necessarily an overt lie, and it's something the woman with dementia can relate to; in her reality, this makes sense.

Most experts agree that the truth should always be the intent. Simply avoiding an unpleasant reaction isn't a good enough reason to lie. Likewise, a lie shouldn't be told just because it's more convenient. But for people who can't make sense of the truth — and in situations in which the truth will cause harm or distress — a therapeutic fib may be the better option.

PLANNING FOR THE HOLIDAYS

The holiday season may loom heavily when you have a loved one living with dementia. By adjusting your expectations and modifying some traditions, you may find meaningful ways to celebrate holidays. Consider these strategies.

Create a calm and safe space

Avoid blinking holiday lights, large displays or decorations that require you to rearrange a familiar room. Avoid safety hazards such as burning candles, fragile decorations or decorations that could be mistaken for edible treats, such as artificial fruits. If you have a tree, secure it to a wall.

Make preparations together

If you bake, your loved one may be able to measure flour, stir batter, roll dough or whatever tasks match current retained skills. You may find it meaningful to open holiday cards or wrap gifts together. The outcome may not be a perfectly wrapped gift or an award-winning pie, but a pleasurable activity is very possible.

Adapt holiday activities

Host a small gathering that's quiet and relaxed. Choose a time that is best for your loved one and keep the rest of the day's routines in place if possible. If you're having guests over, provide a quiet place where your loved one can go for alone time or to visit with one person at a time. If you'll be attending a holiday gathering outside the home, plan to be brief or be prepared to leave early if necessary. Make sure there's a place to rest or take a break. In a facility, celebrate with a small family gathering in the setting that's most familiar to your loved one.

Care for yourself
Use positive self-talk, mindfulness and self-compassion to reduce stress and improve well-being. Turn to Chapter 7 to learn more about these and other practices to help improve your mindset during the holidays — and every day.

In addition, manage your expectations you set for yourself with these tips:
- **Pick and choose.** Decide which holiday activities and traditions are most important. Remember that you can't do it all. Focus on what you enjoy.
- **Simplify.** Bake fewer cookies. Ask others to help by providing parts of holiday meals. Use disposable plates and utensils.
- **Delegate.** Remember family members and friends who have offered their assistance. Let them help with cleaning, writing cards and shopping for gifts. Ask if one of your children or a close friend can stay with your loved one while you go to a holiday party.
- **Trust your instincts.** Resist pressure to celebrate the way others may expect you to. By planning and setting firm boundaries, you can enjoy the pleasures of the season.

offers "Creative Care Imagination Kit: A TimeSlips Engagement Resource," which includes cards with questions, thoughtful actions and story prompts.

Say you're visiting with someone with dementia and, looking out the window, you spot a bird in a tree. Your conversation may go something like this:

You: What do you see?
Response: A bird.

You: Do you want to give it a name?
Response: Robin.

You: What sounds do you imagine it makes?

Asking open-ended questions like these allows you to shift away from depending on memory and instead harness the power and freedom of imagination. This approach is designed to allow for greater engagement and to connect people with their loved ones who are living with dementia.

Focus on feelings

Sometimes, even the best attempts to understand what someone with dementia is saying will fail. If you can't understand what your loved one is trying to communicate, you may not know how to help. In these cases, empathy and reassurance go a long way.

If someone with dementia shows signs of distress and you don't know why or what to do, keep the nonverbal skills you've read about in mind. Stay fully present in a way that shows you care. If it seems OK, touch the person's hand, arm or shoulder. Make sure your body language and facial expressions communicate concern and caring and that you're affirming the person's reality. Communicate with words that affirm the feelings you're noticing. For example, you might say, "I'm sorry you're feeling sad (angry, frustrated)," then offer a reassuring message, like, "I'm here for you," or "I care about you."

These strategies validate a person's emotions and support well-being. Although you may be tempted to skip this step and move toward redirecting or distracting the person, you likely won't achieve the outcome you're hoping for. In most cases, it's only after you validate the person's feelings and reality that your redirection can succeed. Having feelings acknowledged, whether they're good or bad, is a universal need. Sometimes it's all that's needed.

5

Creating a dementia-friendly environment

The best living environment for people with dementia is one that helps them feel calm and happy and helps them maintain the highest level of independence possible. Being in an environment that feels familiar is important for people living with dementia. Simple changes to the home environment can have a positive impact on emotional well-being and independence.

Take some time to look at your home with an eye toward well-being and safety. Dementia can impair judgment, sense of balance, sensory perception and problem-solving skills. These challenges can increase your loved one's risk of injury during daily activities. Start by thinking about your loved one's behavior, abilities and health. Is nighttime wandering common? What about falls? Are stairs a challenge? Then check each room for potential hazards and make note of them. It might also be helpful to request an occupational therapy referral for a home safety evaluation. This offers an objective view of your home.

Once you have a sense of potential safety concerns, you can make simple changes to help your loved one feel more at ease and avoid injury. Here are some tips to consider now or in the future.

EVALUATE LIGHTING

Good lighting can help reduce glare, shadows and reflections. Lighting is especially important on stairs and for the toilet. Night-lights in hallways and near the toilet can help a person with dementia find the bathroom at night.

USE CONTRASTING COLORS; LIMIT BUSY PATTERNS

The use of color and contrast can be helpful for people with dementia, but it's best to avoid heavily patterned wallpaper and fabric.

REDUCE THE RISK OF FALLS

Avoid throw rugs, extension cords and any clutter that can cause your loved one to trip. In particular, ensure that areas where your loved one walks are free of furniture and cords. If the person you're caring for gets up at night, use night-lights in the bedroom, bathroom and hallways.

Install light switches at the top and bottom of stairs. Make sure stairs have at least one handrail that extends beyond the first and last step and consider marking the edges of indoor and outdoor steps with bright tape.

ADD SIMPLE SIGNS

Consider putting signs such as "bowls" or "socks" on cupboards and drawers. Other signs, such as arrows pointing to rooms or a picture of a toilet on the bathroom door, can also be helpful.

REMOVE CLUTTER

This will help the person with dementia find items and not feel overstimulated. Arrange furniture simply and consistently to keep the environment familiar.

REDUCE NOISE

Be aware of sounds coming from the television, radio and kitchen. Too many sounds can add to confusion and contribute to agitation.

AVOID BATHROOM INJURIES

Install a shower chair as well as grab bars near the toilet, near the bathtub and in the shower. Place nonskid strips in the bathtub and shower and on slippery floor surfaces, such as near the bathtub, shower, toilet and sink. Remove plug-in appliances to avoid the risk of electric shock.

PREVENT BURNS OR FIRE

Make sure food isn't too hot and set your water-heater temperature to no higher than 120 degrees Fahrenheit. Avoid using portable space heaters in the bedroom, and keep the controls for electric blankets or heating pads out of reach. If your loved one is a smoker, keep matches or lighters under your control and make sure your loved one never smokes alone. Keep a first-aid kit, a fire extinguisher and working smoke alarms in the home.

PUT AWAY POTENTIALLY DANGEROUS ITEMS

Install locks on cabinets that contain medicine, alcohol, guns, toxic cleaning substances, dangerous utensils and tools. Remove knobs or install safety knobs on the stove, and disconnect the garbage disposal.

TAKE PRECAUTIONS IN THE GARAGE AND BEYOND

Lock all vehicles and consider locking the doors to the garage, shed and basement. Make sure there are working locks on all windows and front and back doors. Keep a spare set of house keys outside the house, in case your loved one locks you out. If needed, install dead bolts high or low on outside doors to make it harder for your loved one to wander out of the house.

If you have a swimming pool or hot tub, install a fence around it with a locked gate. If you have an outdoor grill, remove fuel sources and other equipment when not in use.

SUPPORT DAILY TASKS

An empathetic and flexible approach can help you support daily tasks such as bathing, dressing, using the bathroom and eating. Depending on the stage of dementia, the person in your care may need a little bit of assistance or a lot of help with these everyday activities. If you're providing this type of care, balance the loss of

IF YOUR LOVED ONE WANDERS

Although the term *wandering* is often used for people with dementia, the term suggests that there's no purpose to the person's walking, which is not usually the case. There is almost always a reason why someone with dementia wants to walk, pace or wander. Your loved one might be searching for an item, a person or a location. Or it could be that the person is bored and wants to release some energy.

Some people living with dementia try to follow past routines, such as going to work or the grocery store. But they can get lost even in familiar places because dementia affects the parts of the brain important for visual guidance and navigation. Simply having a diagnosis of dementia doesn't automatically mean that someone can't cross the road safely or take a walk around the block. Some can, and some can't.

Consider these suggestions if you feel your loved one shouldn't walk alone.

Provide supervision
Identify a walking partner. Consider arranging for this person at the times of day when your loved one's desire to walk is highest. Avoid leaving the person with dementia alone in a new or changed environment or in a car.

Install alarms and locks
Various devices can alert you that your loved one is on the move. You might place pressure-sensitive alarm mats at the door or at the person's bedside, put

warning bells on doors, use childproof covers on doorknobs or install an alarm system that chimes when a door is opened. If the person tends to unlock doors, install sliding bolt locks that aren't readily visible.

Camouflage doors

Place removable curtains over doors. Cover doors with paint or wallpaper that matches the surrounding walls. Or place a scenic poster on the door or a sign that says "Stop" or "Do not enter."

Keep keys out of sight

If your loved one is no longer driving, hide the car keys. Also put away shoes, coats, hats and other items that might be associated with leaving home.

Ensure a safe return

Have the person carry an identification card or wear a medical bracelet, and place labels in the person's garments. Also, consider enrolling in the MedicAlert and Alzheimer's Association safe-return program. For a fee, participants receive an identification bracelet, necklace or clothing tags and access to 24-hour support in case of emergency. You also might have your loved one wear a GPS or other tracking device.

If your loved one wanders, search the immediate area for no more than 15 minutes and then contact local authorities and the safe-return program (if you've enrolled). The sooner you seek help, the sooner your loved one is likely to be found.

privacy and independence with respect and empathy. The best approach is one in which you are *doing with* rather than *doing for*. Consider these strategies.

Bathing

Make accommodations that improve the bathing experience for a person living with dementia. You can improve the experience when you:

- **Help your loved one feel in control.** Allow your loved one to do as much as possible. Sometimes all you need to do is get the process started by turning on the shower, filling the bathtub or setting out the soap and washcloth. Ask your loved one's permission as much as you can. For example, you may ask, "Would it be OK if I wash your back while you hold the water nozzle?" Also, let your loved one know what you are about to do next.
- **Make it comfortable.** Have everything, such as towels and shampoo, ready ahead of time and within reach. Soft music or calming scents may be nice.
- **Align with your loved one's preferences.** Some people prefer showers, while others prefer tub baths. Time of day is often important as well. Experiment with morning, afternoon and evening bathing.
- **Keep it private.** If your loved one is self-conscious about being naked, provide a towel for cover when getting in and out of the shower or tub.
- **Dry the person while seated** to reduce fear of falling.
- **Pick your battles.** Bathing once or twice a week can be enough. A sponge rinse at the sink may be good enough.

Dressing

Changes caused by dementia can make dressing a more complicated task for persons living with dementia. Promote independence while offering support by:

- **Not taking over.** Allow the person to do as much as possible, even if the result isn't exactly as you prefer.
- **Making it easy and comfortable.** Choose clothes that are comfortable and easy for the person with dementia to put on and take off independently. Garments that are stretchable, shoes that slip on and clothing that fastens in the front are all good options.
- **Offering choices while limiting options.** Sometimes just a couple of options can help ease frustration. For example, ask, "Do you prefer the red shirt or the floral sweater?" or "Would you like to wear the green shorts or the plaid shorts?" Emptying closets and drawers of clothes that are no longer needed or appropriate can help too.
- **Providing direction.** Set out or hand out pieces of clothing one at a time, starting with what is put on first. As needed, give simple, step-by-step instructions for getting dressed.
- **Being patient.** Rushing the dressing process rarely makes things go faster or easier.
- **Picking your battles.** If your loved one always wants to wear the same thing, buy more than one of the outfits, if possible.

Toileting

As dementia progresses, toileting independence and issues with incontinence are not uncommon. Help your loved one maintain a sense of dignity by:
- **Promoting independence.** Consider raising the toilet seats and installing grab bars. Help as needed, using verbal cues such as reminding them to pull down their pants and visual cues such as handing them toilet paper or having it located within easy eyesight.
- **Making the bathroom easy to find.** A sign on the door that says "Toilet" may be helpful. You can even use a picture of a toilet.

- **Staying alert for signs.** Restlessness or tugging on clothing may signal the need to use the bathroom.
- **Establishing a schedule.** Provide bathroom breaks on a regular schedule, such as every two hours and before meals, bathing or other activities.
- **Being proactive.** To help prevent nighttime accidents, limit certain types of fluids — such as those with caffeine — in the evening.
- **Offering support.** When accidents happen, take them in stride. Use encouraging words and avoid criticism.

Mealtimes

Most people living with dementia can continue to manage and enjoy mealtimes. In the later stages, assistance may be needed. Help ensure the best possible experience and proper nutrition with:
- **Routine.** Schedule meals around the same time every day as much as possible. If mealtimes are too long or difficult, consider frequent, smaller meals throughout the day.
- **Hydration.** Offer fluids throughout the day to promote adequate hydration. Food with high water content, such as fruit, soups, milkshakes and smoothies, can also help.
- **A calm environment.** Distractions at mealtime can create agitation. To reduce distractions, turn off the TV or radio. Remove unnecessary clutter from the table. Silence phones.
- **Easy-to-use dishes and utensils.** Consider solid-colored instead of patterned dishes, bowls instead of plates, spoons instead of forks or fingers instead of utensils. Bendable straws or lidded cups may be useful.
- **A nonslip placemat.** To make sure plates or bowls don't slip around, consider setting them on a placemat with traction. You can make your own nonslip placemat from a roll of the rubbery mesh typically used to line shelves. Even a damp washcloth will work.

- **Simple servings.** Cut food into bite-size pieces before serving, or make finger foods. Serve one type of food at a time, as deciding what to eat may be agitating.
- **Healthful variety.** Make favorite and familiar foods, while ensuring generous servings of vegetables, fruits and whole grains.
- **Encouragement and modeling.** You can help with the basic mechanics of eating by eating with your loved one as a way of demonstrating how to hold a spoon, when to take a drink or how to chew enough after a bite. Gently hold your loved one's hand to help with using a utensil.
- **Shared meals.** Eat together when possible and treat mealtimes as an opportunity to visit.
- **Dental care.** Regular dental care can help prevent problems that make eating painful.

Medications

Part of your role as a care partner may be to ensure that the person with dementia is properly taking all medications. This is no easy feat, especially if your loved one needs help in this area.

It's a good idea to keep a record of all medications your loved one is taking, including all prescription and nonprescription medicines and supplements such as vitamins or herbal remedies. Record how much and how often each medication should be taken and the health care provider who prescribed or recommended it. You may also want to list any allergies to medications or past medications that caused difficult side effects.

Be sure to share this list with your loved one's pharmacist and bring it to medical appointments to check for potential drug interactions. It's important that all members of your loved one's health care team be aware

A NUTRITIONAL CHECKUP

Good nutrition is critical to health and well-being. It's especially important for older adults, including those with dementia. Over time, poor nutrition (malnutrition) in older adults can weaken muscle and bone, affecting mobility and increasing the risk of falls. Malnutrition also weakens the immune system, making it harder for the body to heal from injuries and increasing the risk of illness. Poor nutrition in older adults may lead to hospitalization, longer hospital stays after surgery and even death. In particular, low protein in a diet can negatively affect the eyes, kidneys, brain and other organs. In people living with dementia, poor nutrition may make challenging behaviors worse.

The risk of malnutrition increases as the dementia progresses, especially once the person needs help to eat. Be on the lookout for these common causes of malnutrition in a person with dementia.

Pain
Poorly fitted dentures, gum infections, cavities and other dental problems can make eating painful.

Diminished sense of taste and smell
These senses often decline later in life, robbing food of much of its flavor.

Failure to recognize food as food
Some people with dementia don't realize that items on a plate are food and aren't sure if they should eat them.

Medications

Certain drugs commonly prescribed for older adults can affect the appetite: for example, antibiotics and certain medications for depression, heart failure, high blood pressure and osteoporosis.

Poor chewing and swallowing skills

In later stages of the disease, a person with dementia will likely have difficulty chewing and swallowing.

Reduced social contact

Another contributor to malnutrition is social isolation — and the loneliness and depression that can go along with it. Social contact has a positive effect on eating well and increases morale and well-being, factors that contribute to appetite.

Malnutrition is a complex problem, but even small changes make a big difference in an older person's health and well-being. The mealtime strategies on pages 86-87 are a good place to start. Don't forget that healthy adults — including care partners — need good nutrition too.

If you're concerned that you or your loved one isn't getting proper nutrition, talk to your loved one's care team. They can offer guidance on the use of vitamins or supplemental beverages, healthy and simple meal planning and other strategies to support eating skills.

of the medications the person is taking, especially when prescribing new medications.

Even with all this information at your fingertips, your loved one's loss of short-term memory may present challenges. Forgetting to take or taking too much of a medication is common among people living with dementia. To prevent these and other problems, consider these tips:

- **Use memory aids.** Reminder notes, calendars or lists can help your loved one know when to take medications.
- **Establish a daily routine.** Create and stick to a medication schedule, such as taking medications first thing in the morning, at mealtime or before going to sleep at night.
- **Use a pill dispenser.** Organize medications using a seven-day pill dispenser, or buy a pill dispenser with reminder alarms.
- **Ask your pharmacist about blister packs.** Your local or online pharmacy may be able to presort daily doses of medications into blister packs. You or your loved one can then punch out each day's medications one day at a time.
- **Set reminder alerts.** Program alarms on your loved one's watch or ask another family member to call at appropriate times with friendly reminders.
- **Install locks.** Use locks on any cabinets containing prescription and nonprescription medications to limit access.
- **Check dates on bottles and packaging.** Remove outdated or discontinued medications from the home.

In more advanced stages of dementia, you'll likely become more involved in your loved one's medication regimen. When giving a medication, explain in simple language what the medicine is for and how it should be taken. Try to avoid power struggles. If your loved one is unwilling to take a medication, consider taking a break and trying again later. If swallowing pills become difficult, ask your provider or pharmacist if the medication comes in liquid form. Or ask if you can safely crush the medication and mix it with food, such as pudding or applesauce.

REDUCE LATE-DAY CONFUSION AND IMPROVE SLEEP

As daylight fades and evening begins, your loved one may become confused, anxious, agitated and irritable. *Sundowning* is a label that's been associated with these symptoms. Although sundowning has been studied for several decades, its cause remains unclear. However, certain factors seem to contribute, such as changes to the body's circadian clock, low lighting, disruption in routine, poor sleep, medications wearing off, low energy reserves at the end of the day and boredom.

What you can do

If your loved one is experiencing increased agitation or confusion later in the day, you can help lessen these symptoms and help your loved one get better sleep. Consider these suggestions:

- **Stick to a routine.** Try to maintain a predictable schedule for bedtime, waking, meals and activities. Try to incorporate regular and predictable activities later in the day.
- **Avoid late-afternoon appointments.** If possible, schedule medical appointments and other outings in the morning or early afternoon. In a strange or unfamiliar setting, bring familiar items — such as photographs — to create a more relaxed, familiar setting.

- **Encourage exposure to sunlight.** If your loved one is able, spend some time together outdoors, such as on a walk. Exposure to sunlight during the day can reset a person's internal clock and encourage nighttime sleepiness. Even sitting by a window can help.
- **Limit daytime napping.** Naps can make it harder to fall asleep at night. If your loved one needs rest, keep the naps short and schedule them earlier in the day.
- **Limit caffeine.** Avoid serving coffee, cola or other caffeinated drinks after the morning hours.
- **Avoid or reduce alcohol and nicotine.** These substances can affect a person's ability to sleep.
- **Create a quiet evening atmosphere.** Try to reduce background noise and stimulating activities, including TV viewing, which can sometimes be upsetting. Play familiar gentle music in the evening or relaxing sounds of nature, such as the sound of waves. Or read quietly to your loved one.
- **Minimize shadows.** Close the shades or blinds and keep your home well lit.
- **Notice triggers.** Pay attention to which afternoon and evening activities or routines seem to contribute to sundowning. Replace them with activities that are soothing to your loved one.

As evening falls, watch for signs of confusion or agitation. If you notice sundowning behavior, or if your loved one wakes from sleep in a disoriented state, remain calm, listen and let the person know that everything is OK. Try to address any unmet needs, such as thirst or a full bladder. Avoid arguing or using physical restraint. Allow your loved one to safely pace if needed.

If sundowning behaviors or sleep disturbances are causing distress, talk to your loved one's health care team. An underlying condition, such as a urinary tract infection, restless leg syndrome or sleep apnea, might be worsening sundowning behavior, especially if sundowning develops quickly.

BE COMPASSIONATE TO YOURSELF

I recognize that caregiving is now the major chapter in my life. My future holds other chapters. But for now I'm being remade and reformed by my role of caregiving into a gentler, more compassionate, more patient, kinder person.

This reflection comes from Rosalie, whom you heard from at the start of this chapter. When she wrote this, she had been on her caregiving journey for a number of years.

As you've read many times throughout this book, each care partner's experience is individual; no two are alike. In addition, no care partner should feel the need to become some kind of superhero. For some, like Rosalie, the experience can be transformative, and for others, not so much. Take what makes sense from this chapter and use the strategies that best fit your unique situation.

If you find that there's no solution for the challenges you're facing, turn to self-compassion, a practice you'll learn more about in the next chapter. Sometimes this is all you can give yourself.

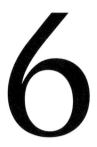

Living well as a caregiver

I was 55; John was 57. The first inkling that something was wrong started with John's ability to drive. Prior to GPS navigation, he could find his way anywhere, with or without a map. He became confused when driving to familiar locations and at stop signs and traffic lights, not stopping — or stopping half a block too soon. John was also experiencing wild dreams — he would twitch, shout, toss and pound on the bed. He'd often say he was fighting off a bear.

We scheduled an appointment with John's doctor. After several days of testing, John was diagnosed with mild cognitive impairment and REM sleep disorder. Feelings of disbelief and fear overwhelmed us.

When we got home, we called our children. I was a basket case. I couldn't sleep or eat. In my head, I went directly from the mild cognitive impairment diagnosis John had received to the final stage of dementia. John

and I have been happy together for years. It's not to say
we've felt that way every day, but on the whole, we
simply love being together. John makes me laugh. I make
him laugh. Would we laugh again? I felt like I was in
quicksand and couldn't find solid ground.

This reflection from Rosalie offers a glimpse into the
very beginning of one person's journey as a care partner.
Becoming a dementia care partner is an unexpected role,
and each care partner experiences this role in a different way. Many factors impact the caregiving experience,
including your relationship with the person you're caring
for, other roles and responsibilities in your life and your
personal coping strategies and social support.

For some, the role of caregiving can feel like a heavy,
ever-increasing load. For others, caregiving is deeply
fulfilling, rewarding and meaningful. Most agree that
being a care partner to someone with dementia is one
of the hardest jobs they've ever had.

According to a recent report, nearly half of all family
caregivers say they feel somewhat stressed, and more than
a third say they're highly stressed. Care partners juggle
many responsibilities. They often feel that their loved ones
are depending on them for help with daily living as well as
for emotional support, comfort and a sense of security.

As a care partner, you're managing these daily demands
while also living with the knowledge that your loved
one has a disease that will worsen over time. You may
have difficulty accepting this and adapting to changes
that are beyond your control. Each change along the
way may feel like a new loss to be mourned.

In the face of these challenges, it's natural to feel a range
of powerful and conflicting emotions. You may feel sad,

angry, guilty, overwhelmed, exhausted or lonely. All these feelings and experiences are to be expected.

You will encounter frustrations and losses. You will make mistakes. Many things won't go the way you'd hoped. But the more you open your heart to this reality instead of fighting against it, the more likely you are to find inner strength and peace.

This chapter offers suggestions for addressing the ups and downs of being a care partner. You'll also learn ways to develop the inner strength you need for the days ahead. The most important thing to remember is that you're not alone. You're part of a large family of dementia care partners — each one unique, but all sharing in the struggle.

MOVING TOWARD ACCEPTANCE

Maybe a loved one was recently diagnosed with dementia and you're struggling to adjust to this life-changing news. Or maybe you thought you'd reached a kind of acceptance, only to feel the rug pulled out from under you when your loved one loses a skill or shows a noticeable decline in memory. Rather than face the uncertainty that comes with a diagnosis or an unwanted change, you may unintentionally be in denial.

On some level, you may be holding out hope that your loved one will stay the same or even get better. You may look for signs that your loved one isn't truly ill, tell yourself that the changes you see are part of the aging process or convince yourself that a good day is a sign that your loved one is improving. You may reject the fact that the disease will significantly affect your relationship. These are all examples of denial and are completely understandable. Anything that makes you feel afraid or vulnerable or threatens your sense of control can cause feelings of denial.

Occasional periods of denial are understandable. In some cases, initial, short-term denial can even be a good thing. It can give you time to adjust to a painful or stressful issue. But a persistent state of denial can be unhealthy. Research shows that when care partners avoid painful emotions and engage in denial and wishful thinking, they experience more stress. Those who accept their situation and allow for the emotions that come with it, in contrast, tend to experience better mental health.

Denying the reality of your situation can keep you from using the tools, skills and support you need. Accepting your situation offers opportunities that can help you and the person living with dementia. This is what makes acceptance so powerful.

Acceptance is a choice to be with your situation just as it is. Developing an attitude of acceptance doesn't mean you're supporting the unfairness of the situation. It simply means that you accept what you can't change. When you're willing to accept things as they are, you're demonstrating humility, courage and compassion — qualities that give you strength.

Acceptance also means giving your full attention to what's happening now. As one care partner said, "I had to stop dwelling on the way my dad used to be and be fully present for who he is today." This is an example of acceptance.

Acceptance is about reality, but it's also a turning point toward change and transformation. Acceptance can lead you down a path toward greater well-being. Following are four ways you can harness the power of acceptance.

Realize that you can't control everything

To find some relief from caregiving stress, try to recognize the difference between what's within your power to change and what isn't. Trying to change something you can't control leads to negative feelings like anger and resentment.

No matter what you do, you can't change your loved one's disease. While you know this on some level, the way you think, feel and respond may be a way of rejecting this basic truth. This is where having realistic expectations can help, like being honest about what you can and can't control.

For example, you can't control how your loved one's disease will progress or whether or not extended family members or friends agree with your decisions. However, you can control your efforts to seek support, the caregiving skills you build and how you choose to respond to a challenging situation.

Over time, many care partners learn to let go of what they can't control, including not being able to "save" someone living with dementia or make the person better. Letting go of the expectation to "fix" someone with dementia can lift a burden from your shoulders. When you don't feel the pressure to fix the things that are out of your control, you may discover that you can engage with your loved one — and yourself — with greater compassion.

Be a good-enough care partner

As dementia progresses, you'll need to offer more help to your loved one. You'll likely take on responsibilities for things you may not have done before, like certain household tasks, yardwork or bill paying. You may also become the primary source of emotional support for the person living with dementia. The person living with dementia will likely be taking cues from you on how to react or what to do next in certain situations.

This is a lot of pressure, especially when you also have your own life to manage.

While you may want to believe that you can do it all — and do it all perfectly — this simply isn't possible. You may also think you need to sacrifice your own needs and be available for your loved one at all times. This isn't healthy for you or for your loved one. These high expectations lead to exhaustion and feelings of guilt. Instead, choose to be a good-enough care partner rather than striving to be great or perfect. Set realistic limits for yourself. Be willing to see any small achievement as a success.

Instead of dwelling on the "shoulds," tell yourself, *I can only do my best, and my best is good enough.*

Forgive yourself

Guilt is often the result of refusing to accept that some things are out of your control. It's helpful to release yourself from that burden by offering yourself forgiveness.

If you were irritated with or critical of someone living with dementia before you knew the diagnosis, forgive yourself. If you made a promise early on to keep someone with dementia living at home but that's no longer the best choice, it's OK. You didn't know then what you know now.

Whether it's making a difficult decision or making a mistake, remember that you're human and you're doing the best you can. No family or care partner can plan for every situation or anticipate every challenge.

There are no perfect families and there are no perfect solutions. This is where self-compassion comes in. Instead of judging and criticizing yourself, be easy on yourself and forgive, even when you're faced with what feels like a personal failing.

Feel what you feel

Your emotions — grief, sadness, anger or all of the above — are a typical part of being a care partner and a human being. All of your emotions provide insight and can help you through tough times.

It's understandable to resent being a caregiver but love the person you're caring for. Rather than label your feelings as bad and push them away, remind yourself that these feelings are natural and even healthy.

This expression of openness toward whatever you're feeling at that moment is actually helpful. Research suggests that being aware and accepting of thoughts and emotions gives them less power and can lessen the stress you feel.

When you're open to noticing negative emotions, without judging them or judging yourself for having them, you're also creating space for positive emotions, like joy or relief, to enter in.

In this way, you're more likely to find greater pleasure in the quiet, unrushed moments, like when you're sitting on the porch with your loved one or sipping a cup of tea at the end of a long day. Feeling joy in life doesn't mean you're not taking your responsibilities seriously. It means you're taking care of yourself.

ADDRESSING GUILT AND GRIEF

Two common emotions that dementia care partners feel are guilt and grief.

Guilt is an expected emotion woven throughout the care partner experience. While guilt can be useful when it pushes you to make amends for something you've done wrong or for harm you've caused others, it's often an undeserved emotion for care partners.

Grief is a deep and sometimes complex emotion people feel when they experience a loss. It's both a universal and a personal experience. For dementia care partners, grief can be an ever-present part of the journey. Here's more on guilt and grief, including ways to cope with both emotions.

How to cope with guilt

As a care partner, you may struggle with guilt for a range of imagined failings:
- Feeling anger or frustration toward the person living with dementia.
- Feeling trapped in the care partner role or wishing the person with dementia wasn't a part of your life.
- Feeling that you fall short in comparison with other care partners.
- Needing a break from your role as a care partner.
- Moving your loved one out of the home and into a care community, like a nursing home.

- Needing help from others and not being able to do everything yourself.
- Feeling that you've failed to meet every one of your loved one's needs perfectly.
- Feeling guilty for experiencing happiness and enjoyment in life.

If, like many other care partners, you're struggling with guilt for these or other reasons, try taking steps toward adopting a more balanced and realistic perspective. Here are several suggestions that can help.

Notice it

Acknowledging that you're feeling guilt is an important first step. If you try to ignore feelings of guilt, you may experience even more negative thoughts and stress. It may sound counterproductive and even unpleasant, but in order to move on from guilt, you first have to acknowledge it. Once you've done that, you can address guilt in a more rational way.

Start by asking yourself, *Am I feeling guilty for things that are outside of my control?* From there, you have several options:
- Forgive yourself and let it go. It will pass if you let it.
- Forgive yourself and make a decision about how you will act in a similar situation next time.
- Forgive yourself and take some action that could benefit yourself or others.

Talk to others

Don't keep your guilt bottled up. Talk to someone who will really listen and understand what you're going through, like a trusted friend or another care partner.

Sharing your feelings with others will help to normalize the feelings and give you a more balanced perspective.

Remember that guilt is common

Many other care partners have likely experienced every reason you can think of to feel guilt. It's natural to experience moments of anger or frustration, to yearn for time away and to need the help and support of others.

Tend to your grief

Some people start to grieve soon after a loved one receives a diagnosis. Others may begin to grieve as the disease progresses or after a loved one has died. You may grieve for the person who is changing and for the changes to your life.

Tending to your grief as a care partner is essential. Grief can weigh you down and show up as anger or depression. Being with your grief can bring a renewed sense of peace and ease to your life. It's a necessary part of the full human experience.

Types of grief

Although the process of grieving differs from person to person, it can be comforting to know that certain experiences are common among care partners. If you've experienced any of these types of grief, you're far from alone.

Disenfranchised grief. Early on, you may struggle with two conflicting realities: On the one hand, your loved one is alive and well and may seem unchanged to family members and friends. On the other hand, you've started to notice small but increasingly frequent changes in your loved one that signal bigger and more painful changes to come.

Without the full understanding and support of those around you, it may seem as if what you're experiencing doesn't matter and that you don't have the right to grieve. This is sometimes called disenfranchised grief.

Ambiguous loss. This type of grief happens when you feel a sense of loss or mourning for someone who's still there physically but mentally and emotionally no longer present in the way you need or want him or her to be. A spouse, parent or friend may be right there in front of you, for example, yet you mourn not being able to share emotional support, cook meals together or talk about the news of the day in the ways that you used to.

Ambiguous loss can vary depending on the type of dementia. In Alzheimer's disease, for example, care partners may experience losses related to changes in thinking and memory, like the ability to have meaning-ful conversations. Behavioral variant frontotemporal degeneration causes someone to lose the ability to have appropriate emotions and empathy for others. This is very painful for care partners and families. And Lewy body dementia can cause fluctuations in thinking that can make it seem as if someone's moving back and forth from one stage of dementia to another, but in reality, these fluctuations happen at every stage of the disease. This can cause a similar back and forth of emotions for care partners and families.

Anticipatory grief. As you learn about dementia and plan for the future, you may become consumed by worries of future changes and challenges and start to grieve losses that haven't happened yet. For example, you may mourn a time when your loved one no longer recognizes you or needs to move out of the home and into a care community. This kind of grief is known as anticipatory grief.

Being with grief

Rather than shove grief aside, allow yourself to acknowledge and feel your grief and the other emotions that can come with it. You may be surprised when strong feelings like anger, guilt, frustration and resentment arise. Try to be with these feelings with openness and kindness.

Know that people may not understand your grief. Most people think grief happens when someone dies. Talk to someone you trust about your feelings. This can be a good friend, another care partner, an understanding professional or a supportive member of your family. For some care partners, support groups can be helpful. Look for a group with whom you feel safe sharing your experience and your emotions.

Because dementia worsens over time, you may experience many moments of loss over time. What triggers your grief may seem small, like the first time you attend a caregiver support group. Or it may feel overwhelmingly big, like the day your loved one enters memory care.

Adjusting to the changes and losses is a process. Like the practice of acceptance, addressing grief happens in several ways. These steps will help you work through your grief in the ways that are best for you.

7

Understanding caregiver stress and burnout

Along with guilt and grief, you may experience stress. Caring for someone living with dementia is emotionally and physically challenging. You may feel that you're constantly on call. And your role can change from day to day, demanding a lot of flexibility. You also may be grieving your loved one's failing health. It's hard to watch someone decline. You may be grieving about the changes to your relationship too.

It's no wonder that caregiver stress is common among dementia care partners. By simply recognizing and understanding caregiver stress, you're taking an important step toward protecting your health and well-being.

Watch for these signs and symptoms of caregiver stress:
- Feeling overwhelmed or constantly worried.
- Often feeling tired or exhausted.
- Getting too much sleep or not enough sleep.

- Gaining or losing weight.
- Becoming easily irritated or angry.
- Having a hard time concentrating.
- Losing interest in activities you used to enjoy.
- Feeling sad.
- Having frequent headaches, bodily pain or other physical problems.
- Misusing alcohol or drugs, including prescription medications.

People who experience caregiver stress, especially over a long period of time, can be vulnerable to changes in their own health. As a care partner, you're more likely to experience symptoms of depression or anxiety. In addition, you might not get enough sleep or physical activity or eat a balanced diet — any of which increases your risk of medical problems, such as heart disease and diabetes.

When caregiver stress is ongoing (chronic), it can lead to burnout or compassion fatigue. Caregiver burnout is sometimes described as a feeling of overload. You may lack energy and enthusiasm for caregiving and other areas of life. You may feel indifferent toward and detached from the person you're supporting. Lacking a sense of meaning or accomplishment is another sign of burnout.

It's important to address caregiver stress, compassion fatigue and burnout. They can affect your health and quality of life, as well as your ability to care for someone else. In the next section, you'll learn about strategies to help you manage stress and nurture your health and well-being. If you're worried about stress or burnout, consider talking to your health care provider, a licensed mental health professional or your loved one's care team. Don't hesitate to seek help for any concerns or symptoms you have.

BALANCE YOUR FOCUS

It's necessary and healthy to notice stress, as well as guilt, grief and other feelings that are distressing or negative. However, it's *not* healthy to focus on negative feelings for so long that they crowd out positive experiences and feelings. For the right balance, it's best to give painful or difficult emotions the attention they need when they come up, but then actively work to embrace positive experiences and emotions.

Embracing the good may be easier said than done. It's easier for the brain to pay attention to bad things and overlook good things. This is a result of how human beings have evolved. For early humans, paying attention to dangerous threats was a matter of life and death. Those who were more attuned to the danger around them were more likely to survive.

ARE YOU AT RISK OF CAREGIVER STRESS AND BURNOUT?

Your risk of caregiver stress and burnout is higher if you:
- Live with or are married to the person you're caring for.
- Are isolated from other people.
- Have depression.
- Are in poor health.
- Are struggling financially.
- Lack coping skills or have trouble solving problems.
- Don't have a choice about being a caregiver.

Today, this focus on the bad is known as *negativity bias*. Research shows that the brain is more active when it's responding to something negative. As a result, the brain tends to be influenced more powerfully by bad news and negative experiences, as opposed to good news and positive experiences. Often, positive experiences pass you by without your even noticing them.

Here's an example of negativity bias: Imagine that you're spending an afternoon with your daughter. You laugh, share stories and enjoy great conversation. You feel truly connected and joyful for this rare time together. As you're about to part ways, your daughter says that she doesn't think you should be taking her dad (your husband) to the adult day program he usually attends. "His dementia isn't that bad," your daughter says. "He doesn't belong there."

You're instantly annoyed. As you drive home, you think about her opinion over and over. By the time you're home, you're angry, exhausted and drained. You feel as if your daughter doesn't appreciate the respite you receive — and need — by taking your husband to the adult day program. You go to bed feeling that the day was ruined.

What happened to all those good feelings from the day? Your positive experiences were drowned out by the negative ones; this is how negativity bias works. In short, the bad emotions carry more weight than the good ones. As a result, you think about the bad experiences for longer periods of time, and they weigh more heavily on you.

Fortunately, you can overcome your negativity bias and focus more on positive emotions by taking the following steps.

Address negative self-talk

Self-talk is the way you talk to yourself in your head. These automatic thoughts can be positive or negative, but more often than not, they're negative. For care partners, negative self-talk may include thoughts of self-doubt and criticism, regret, worry and guilt. Forms of negative self-talk include:

Filtering

This is when you magnify the negative aspects of a situation and filter out all of the positive ones. In the example you just read, you had a great afternoon with your daughter, filled with connection and joy. However, your visit ended with a short conversation in which you had a disagreement. The rest of the day and evening, you focused only on your disagreement and forgot about the wonderful time you spent with your daughter.

Personalizing

This is when something bad happens and you automatically blame yourself. For example, your coffee group canceled its gathering for tomorrow, and you think it's because no one wanted to be around you and hear about your struggles.

Catastrophizing

Automatically believing the worst is going to happen is known as catastrophizing. Maybe you're having a bad morning, and you tell yourself that as long as you're a caregiver, your life is going to be miserable.

Polarizing

Polarizing happens when you see things only as either good or bad, with no middle ground between the two. Maybe you feel like you have to be perfect or you'll be a total failure. For example, if you can't convince your spouse to shower, you tell yourself you're the worst caregiver ever.

Using "should" statements

A "should" statement is when you believe you should think, feel or behave in a certain way. Maybe you feel you *should* be able care for your loved one by yourself or that you *should* keep your promise to not move your loved one to a care community.

It's important to notice when you're engaged in negative self-talk so you can learn to change the pattern. From there, try to explore what's causing the negative feelings. Is your anger stemming from a sense of feeling overwhelmed, scared or lonely? Is it coming from the impossible expectations you've set for yourself or that others have placed on you? Questions like these can help you pause and see your situation in a more balanced way.

The next time a negative conversation starts playing in your head, try asking yourself the following questions:
• Would I talk this way to my good friend?
• What am I really (angry, frustrated, concerned) about?
• Is what I'm angry or worried about just what I'm thinking at this moment? (Remember, thoughts are real, but they are not necessarily true.)
• Do I really need to be concerned or worried about this?
• What will happen if I ignore this?
• Why am I doing this? Is this someone else's expectation?
• Can I settle for a good-enough-for-now solution?

Savor the positive

Because the brain naturally gravitates toward the negative, it's important to give extra time and attention to good things when they happen. While negative experiences can be quickly transferred and stored in the brain, it takes more of an effort to get the same effect with positive and pleasant experiences. When something good happens, take a moment to really focus on it, be with it and savor it. Replay the moment several times and focus on the positive feelings the memory evokes.

What you focus on determines the parts of your brain that strengthen over time. In other words, if you pay more attention to positive or pleasant experiences, no matter how big or small, your brain can be rewired for resilience, optimism, gratitude and positive emotion.

You may find this approach helpful as you look for moments of connection with the person living with dementia, appreciating whatever strengths and abilities remain. Pay attention to any aspect of life that you're grateful for, even if it's simply the ability to enjoy the morning sunrise and sip a cup of your favorite tea.

PRACTICING MINDFULNESS

Mindfulness is a type of meditation in which you focus on being intensely aware of what you're sensing and feeling in the moment, without interpretation or judgment. Practicing mindfulness can help you reduce stress, make better decisions and be truly present with the person living with dementia. It can also enhance your capacity to experience the joys of everyday life. Mindfulness can address the negative impact of caregiver stress and help you be kinder to yourself and others.

A growing body of research shows that mindfulness is helpful for dementia care partners. One study found that people who care for family members with Alzheimer's disease and other dementias were less stressed and their mood was more stable when they practiced a type of meditation called mindfulness-based stress

HOW TO ADOPT A GRATITUDE PRACTICE

Gratitude plays an important role in well-being. For dementia care partners in particular, research shows that adopting a gratitude practice can improve coping skills and relieve feelings of distress.

Here are three ways to start a gratitude practice, from "The Mayo Clinic Handbook for Happiness":

- **Keep a gratitude journal.** Write in it every day. What you write can be as simple as a kind gesture from a stranger at the grocery store. Any positive thoughts or actions count, no matter how small.
- **Use gratitude cues.** Place photos of things or people that make you happy where you'll see them often. Or post positive notes or inspirational quotes on your refrigerator door or by your computer to reinforce feelings of gratitude.
- **Make a gratitude jar.** Keep an empty jar, with scratch paper and a pen next to it, in an accessible place at home. Write one thing you're grateful for on a piece of paper every day and drop it in the jar. Encourage family members to do this too. At some point during the day, take a few notes out of the jar and read them.

reduction (MBSR). Another study suggested that MBSR is more helpful than caregiver education in terms of improving mental health, reducing stress and relieving depression. A more recent review found that MBSR may help with anxiety and depression in people caring for family members with dementia.

Experts believe that mindfulness works, in part, by helping people accept their experiences, including painful emotions, rather than avoid them.

Mindfulness also offers unique benefits for care partners, according to Marguerite Manteau-Rao, a licensed clinical social worker. Manteau-Rao developed the Mindfulness-Based Dementia Care approach to training dementia caregivers at the Osher Center for Integrative Health at the University of California, San Francisco.

In her book, "Caring for a Loved One With Dementia," Manteau-Rao says that mindfulness:
- Helps care partners spend less time in a stressful state of mind, which is usually associated with thinking too much about the past or worrying about a future event or situation.
- Trains care partners to take the time to pause in the heat of a difficult situation.
- Helps care partners to be more aware of the person with dementia, helping them to notice nonverbal signals.
- Helps care partners shift from a rushed, task-driven mode to a state of simply being. This can help the person with dementia feel recognized and respond more positively.
- Promotes a calm, centered presence.
- Increases sensory awareness. This helps care partners anticipate environmental stressors and make appropriate changes that help the person with dementia.

- Teaches ways to connect with and signal to the person with dementia that you're attuned to the person's present state even if the person is no longer able to speak in ways that you can understand.

Use the practices at the end of this chapter to get acquainted with mindfulness.

SHOWING YOURSELF COMPASSION

Self-compassion is closely linked to mindfulness. During the practice of mindfulness, you build a sense of self-awareness around your thoughts, feelings, sensations and surroundings.

Self-compassion is an attitude you can add to your mindfulness experience. It involves being kind to yourself, especially when you are caught up in harsh self-judgment or you feel as if you've failed. Self-compassion helps you remember that all humans are imperfect, and that's OK.

In "The Mindful Self-Compassion Workbook," psychologists Kristin Neff, Ph.D., and Christopher Germer, Ph.D., describe self-compassion in the following ways.

Treating yourself with kindness

When you're feeling low or you're in the midst of a painful situation, talk to yourself the way you would talk to a good friend.

You may tell yourself, *This is really stressful. You're doing your best right now.* Give yourself the kind of support you need to hear most in that moment.

Accepting that humans are flawed

Rather than beat yourself up for what you see as imperfections, remind yourself that all humans are imperfect. Everyone experiences failure and a sense of not being good enough at times. Acknowledge your failures and imperfections with nonjudgmental compassion. Remind yourself, *I'm flawed, and that's what makes me like everyone else.*

THE STOP PRACTICE

In addition to formally scheduling a time and a place to practice mindfulness, you can practice mindfulness during everyday activities, like when you're stopped at a red light in your car, washing your hands or sitting down to eat a meal. One way to do this is with a practice developed by Jon Kabat-Zinn, Ph.D., called STOP.

This practice helps you to take a brief step back from the stressors of the day and the worries that may be circulating in your mind. It brings you back into the present so you can regain perspective and better regulate your response to pressure.

First, identify various activities you do regularly throughout the day. Any of the activities listed above are good examples. Use these activities as cues to pause. This practice can help you reduce your stress and invite more

Being mindful of negative thoughts and feelings

You've already learned that paying attention to your thoughts can help you respond more effectively to difficult emotions and situations. This kind of mindfulness is also a key element of self-compassion. Instead of resisting or pushing away negative thoughts, feelings and sensations, let them be and acknowledge them as something that's momentary and passing.

calm into your day. Over time, STOP may become a habit and a consistent part of your mindfulness practice.

Here's how it works:
- **S** Stop. Whatever you're doing, just pause momentarily.
- **T** Take a few breaths.
- **O** Observe your thoughts. Where has your mind gone? You may notice that you are engaging in a lot of negative self-talk. What do you feel? Research shows that just naming your emotions can turn the volume down and have a calming effect. What is happening around you? Observe your surroundings.
- **P** Proceed and resume your activities, or use what you've learned during this practice to change course.

Self-compassion is essential to health and well-being. The first step toward believing that you can be a compassionate care partner is to be compassionate and caring toward yourself.

THE SELF-COMPASSION BREAK

Like STOP, a practice called the self-compassion break from Kristin Neff, Ph.D., can help you be kinder to yourself. You can use it anytime, but it can be especially helpful when you're facing difficult or painful situations.

Here's how it works:

1. Acknowledge what you're feeling and tell yourself, *This is a moment of suffering.* Instead of the word *suffering*, you may use the word *painful* or any other word that feels right to you.

2. Tell yourself, *I am not alone. We all struggle and feel pain and suffering.*

3. Put your hands over your heart. Feel the warmth of your hands and their gentle touch on your chest. If there's another soothing touch that feels right for you, use that instead.

4. Say one of the following to yourself:
   - May I be kind to myself.
   - May I give myself the compassion I need.
   - May I forgive myself.
   - May I be patient.
   - May I feel ease.
   - May I remember that I am enough.

MINDFULNESS BREATHING PRACTICE

Focusing your attention on your breath is a common mindfulness practice. Since your breath is always in the present, this practice becomes a way to stay in, as well as return to, the present moment.

1. Find a comfortable position, seated on a chair or on the floor on a cushion. Your eyes may be open or closed; you may find it easier to maintain your focus if your eyes are closed.

2. Take three full breaths in and out. Then return to your natural breathing.

3. Tune in to your natural breath. Feel the natural flow of your breath — in and then out. You don't need to change anything about how you breathe. Notice where you feel your breath in your body; it may be in your belly, or you may notice it in your chest, throat or nostrils. Become aware and curious about the breath, noticing its pattern, sounds and any other sensations.

4. When you find that your mind has wandered and you're no longer paying attention to your breath, stop and gently guide your focus back to your breath.

5. Practice this exercise for five to 15 minutes. Follow your breath, notice when the mind wanders and then return back to the breath, over and over. The intention is not to stop the mind from wandering but to notice when your mind wanders so you can bring it back to the breath.

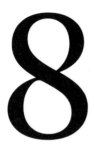

Finding support

Practicing acceptance means that there will be times when you'll need assistance beyond what you alone will be able to provide your loved one. But asking for help may not come easily. You may worry that your loved one won't feel comfortable with other people. Or maybe you think no one else can provide care as well as you can.

The truth is, receiving help can make being a care partner less burdensome, both physically and emotionally. The right assistance can offer resources and skills that you may not have and give you a chance to recharge your batteries. This boost can help you be a more effective, patient and compassionate care partner.

Sources of support fall under two broad categories: informal and formal. Here's how they differ, as well as examples of these two valuable sources of support.

INFORMAL SUPPORT

Informal support includes family, friends, neighbors and faith communities. These groups often consist of people who knew your loved one before the onset of the disease. You may count on them, for example, to make visits or take the person you're caring for to an activity. Their visits may be as valuable for you as they are for the person living with dementia because they keep you both socially connected.

Although these informal sources of support are well meaning, some care partners say that over time, they can drift away, leaving care partners without the support they need. To maintain your connection with the people in your informal support network, be as specific as you can about the help you need.

Through a phone call, letter, email or personal visit, talk to them about the diagnosis as well as the symptoms and changes you're seeing in the person living with dementia. Also let them know the ways in which the person is still very much the same and what things the person with dementia continues to enjoy. Describe your current needs for assistance and offer specific suggestions for the kinds of activities that may be helpful during visits.

Prepare a list of things that routinely need doing and let the people in your informal support network choose tasks that are right for them. Or you may take a different approach, listing the routine tasks you do in a typical day and assigning these tasks to certain individuals on the basis of their qualities and the resources they can provide. Family and friends often find it rewarding to help — it's a way to show they care.

FORMAL SUPPORT

Formal support includes any nonprofit or for-profit agency that provides assistance to individuals in caregiving roles. Home health agencies, community programs like classes, day programs and eldercare centers are all examples. Formal support also includes support groups.

A support group typically consists of other care partners in situations like yours. Support groups meet regularly to share experiences and emotions. Meetings are usually led by a professional or a trained volunteer.

Attending a support group can offer an opportunity for you to hear from others who have dealt with issues like the ones you've experienced. There may also be times when you aren't looking for new ideas or advice — you just want to be among people who understand what you're going through and can relate. Support groups come in many varieties.

TIPS FOR ENLISTING SUPPORT

When someone says, "Let me know if you need something," consider this list as a starting point:
- Provide transportation to doctor appointments.
- Call or visit once a week.
- Help organize and process medical bills.
- Provide a meal.
- Take care of shopping or other errands.
- Do housecleaning, laundry or yardwork.
- Ask occasionally about how I'm doing.
- Be a listener.

Disease-specific groups

These can be groups for care partners of people with dementia, but they can be more specific, like a group for Lewy body dementia or frontotemporal degeneration care partners.

Relationship-specific groups

These groups might bring together people in specific caregiving situations or relationships. Examples include people caring for a spouse or partner, adult children caring for a parent or men who are caregivers.

Peer-led support groups

These groups are led by current or former care partners who share the same experience of caregiving.

Groups led by a trained facilitator

These groups may be led by a social worker, wellness coach, clergyperson, eldercare provider or another professional.

Online and telephone caregiver groups

These groups offer support to people who can't travel to a face-to-face meeting or who need to talk to someone during off hours. You may find a variety of chat rooms, blogs and support groups on the internet. Today, more support groups meet virtually, giving people more options with fewer barriers.

Use your own good judgment about the internet or get recommendations from a trusted medical professional.

COPING WITH FAMILY CONFLICT

Family can be an invaluable source of comfort and support, but it can also be a source of tension. When a family member is diagnosed with dementia, the effect on your entire family can be overwhelming. There are many decisions to make about treatment, care, living arrangements, finances and end-of-life care. As a result, family conflicts are common.

Your family also has its own history of relationships, roles and challenges that can affect how individuals react to a diagnosis and how members see their roles in providing care and support. The following strategies can promote cooperation and lessen family conflicts.

Share responsibility

Make a list of current and anticipated roles and responsibilities. It's unlikely that you'll divide caregiving evenly, but a thorough list will help you consider roles that match each family member's preferences, resources, abilities and emotional capacity.

Some family members might provide hands-on care or make arrangements for the loved one to move in with them. Others might be responsible for respite care, household chores or errands. Your family might designate someone to handle financial or legal issues. One person might research care facilities.

Meet regularly

Hold family meetings to discuss care and other relevant issues. By meeting regularly, such as monthly, you can address a few concerns at a time, avoid getting over-loaded with long meetings, and be more prepared for any changes in care. These can be done in person or via phone or video conference.

Invite everyone who's part of the caregiving team, including family friends and other close contacts. When appropriate, such as with concerns about in-home care, include the family member living with dementia. If you can't resolve disagreements, consider inviting a social worker or clergy member to help facilitate a meeting.

Before you meet, create an agenda and share it. Make it clear that the goal of a meeting is to evaluate care and needs, identify problems and consider solutions. Be open to compromise and possibilities you hadn't considered.

End family meetings with a clear understanding of what has been agreed upon, what each person has agreed to do and what needs to be addressed in the future. You might create a summary of a meeting or an audio recording for family members who can't attend.

Don't criticize

There are many right ways to provide care. Respect each caregiver's abilities, style and values. Be especially supportive of family members responsible for daily, hands-on care.

Communicate honestly

Talk about your feelings in an open, constructive manner during family meetings and informal conversations. If you're angry or stressed, say so. Express your feelings without blaming or shaming anyone else by using "I" statements.

For example, you might say, "I'm feeling overwhelmed with juggling my own schedule and Dad's appointments," rather than, "You don't understand what it's like to manage Dad's schedule." Listen to other family members' feelings too. Listening to others is as important as sharing your feelings.

ADDRESSING CHANGES WITHIN THE FAMILY

When you become a care partner, the relationship within the family system can change and sometimes become strained. This may leave you feeling resentful. Rather than feeling trapped by these circumstances, look for ways to communicate and express your feeling and needs. For example, it may be helpful to:

- Hold regular meetings to update family members about your loved one's condition and the challenges that both of you face.
- Listen closely and respond to family questions, but at the same time, make sure your voice is heard.
- Provide family members with opportunities to help if they're willing to do so. Create a list of your needs and your loved one's needs. Work with family members to delegate tasks, but only to an extent they're comfortable with.
- Consider inviting family members to an in-person or virtual meeting to discuss your needs, as well as

Consider counseling

Even with effective communication and cooperation among family caregivers, you may need help resolving conflicts or coping with stress. You might join a support group for dementia caregivers, seek family counseling or ask for advice from your medical care team. Working through conflicts can help you move on to more important things — caring for your loved one and enjoying your time together.

your loved one's wishes, financial situation and costs of future care. Some families find it helpful to include a professional financial adviser who can guide the meeting. You'll find suggestions for professional advisers later in this book. Encourage questions and suggestions. Invite family members to review their own financial resources. Give them time to decide if they're able to provide financial assistance and, if so, how much.

- Be open about the disease with young children and teenagers. They deserve explanations for the physical and behavioral changes they may be seeing.

Some families find it helpful to meet with a social worker, psychologist, nurse or other professional with specific knowledge about the disease. These specialists can assist you in planning for the future, identifying needs and making decisions.

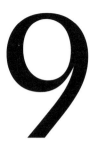

9

Planning for the end of life

Jim loved to garden and enjoyed mowing his lawn. In the days before his death, Jim had his hands in the soil in the raised flower beds he tended. The staff at his assisted living facility brought in grass cuttings so he could feel and smell the grass that brought him so much comfort. Jim died with his family surrounding him and his grandchildren playing on the floor beside him.

For many people, it's not easy to talk about death and dying. But conversations about these topics are incredibly important, not just for someone with a terminal illness but for everyone. When someone is diagnosed with a condition that has an uncertain future, it's especially important to prepare for the end of life in ways that will honor an individual's values, preferences and wishes. It's difficult to know what someone wants at the end of life without talking about it ahead of time.

Talking about death and dying early on allows an individual the opportunity to have more control over care, helps families make important decisions and helps make the transition a little easier for everyone involved. Dementia makes these conversations even more critical — and more difficult.

In the later stages of dementia, a person's ability to think and share thoughts may be compromised. This makes it harder for someone with dementia to express personal wishes. In turn, not knowing a person's preferences makes a difficult situation more challenging and stressful for loved ones. For these reasons, planning for the best possible end-of-life experience, sooner rather than later, is critical. These conversations should include the person with dementia, care providers and loved ones.

Research shows that end-of-life conversations and advance care planning that's done soon after someone is diagnosed with dementia are positive and empowering, both for people living with dementia and their care partners. In this chapter, you'll learn how to have these important conversations.

STARTING THE CONVERSATION

If you're supporting someone with dementia, you may feel unsure about starting a conversation about end-of-life care. Or you may worry about how your loved one will react when you bring up the topic.

Rest assured that starting this conversation is an important way to show someone with dementia that you care. In fact, surveys show that most people *want* to talk about their end-of-life preferences and wish that loved ones would start the conversation.

Starting this conversation shows that you share your loved one's concerns and worries. It also shows that you'll honor and respect your loved one's wishes as much as possible — especially if your loved one can no longer make decisions.

While surveys show that most people find it important to talk about end-of-life care and want to talk about their wishes, these conversations don't always go smoothly. Long before you start this conversation, it can help to make sure that your loved one feels comfortable talking about these important and sensitive issues with you.

For example, when a person with dementia expresses fear, sadness or loss about not being able to do certain things, this can be a natural opening to talk more about these feelings. Talking about feelings early on establishes trust and connection that can help you discuss end-of-life wishes later on. If a family member has recently declined in health or died, this may also open up an opportunity to reflect on that person's care or the circumstances around the death. This may help guide the conversation around what care a person may want — or may not want — near the end of life.

Even with this groundwork, it can be hard to know when and how to talk about the end of life. Adjusting your conversation style and content can help.

For example, depending on the person and the type of dementia, open-ended questions may be too vague. Instead, you may need to ask a question and then offer options or choices. You may also want to start the conversation at a time when the person with dementia is doing well with remembering things, such as distant memories. In this way, you could reflect on the death of a friend or a family member.

Try to understand the whole person by having conversations that explore the person's values, beliefs and preferences. Knowing a person's values can help you make decisions in the future in the event that a person's exact wishes aren't clear. It can also be helpful to have several conversations over a period of time and keep them short and simple.

Above all, make it clear that talking about the end of life is as much for you as it is for your loved one. This goes a long way in establishing a caring connection that allows you to have this important conversation.

Issues to consider

Advance care planning is a dynamic process that involves discussing and documenting an individual's wishes, values and preferences around care and treatment. These discussions are held between an individual and the individual's family members and care providers. Even people who are healthy can — and should — engage in advance care planning. It's never too soon to make an advance care plan.

Advance care planning involves:
- Sharing personal values with loved ones and care providers.
- Getting information on different types of life-sustaining treatments.
- Deciding what types of treatment an individual would want or not want after being diagnosed with a life-limiting illness or at the end of life.
- Completing useful documents that put an individual's care preferences into writing in the event that the individual can no longer articulate them.

This may also be a good opportunity to consider funeral and burial plans. Burial versus cremation, choosing a final resting place and details about a funeral or memorial service are all helpful topics to discuss. Choosing a brain autopsy or a brain donation may be part of this process; these decisions may affect when and how arrangements are made after death.

ADVANCE CARE PLANNING: QUESTIONS TO ASK

- What makes your life worth living? What does a good day look or feel like?
- Which is more important, your quality of life or how long you live?
- What does quality of life mean to you? Does it mean being able to care for yourself? Does it mean recognizing others?
- Whom do you want to make decisions for you if you can't speak for yourself? Examples include your spouse or partner, an adult child or a trusted friend.
- Would you want life-sustaining measures in the last stages of dementia or as you're dying? For example, would you want CPR if your heart stopped beating?
- Where do you want to spend your last days if you're ill? At home? At a nursing home? In a hospital?
- If you knew your life was coming to an end, what would bring you comfort and make dying feel safe? Whom would you want to be with you?
- What are your beliefs about the end of life? How do you want them to be respected and honored?

PUTTING PREFERENCES IN WRITING

After having these conversations, it's important to document the answers to these questions. This is where advance directives can help.

Living wills and other advance directives are written, legal instructions that spell out your preferences for medical care if you're unable to make decisions for yourself. These documents help people with dementia and their care partners make decisions about end-of-life care. These documents — and the conversations around them — help make sure that a person's wishes are spelled out and honored.

In the U.S., each state has different forms and requirements for creating advance directives, but they all must be in writing. The documents may also need to be signed by a witness or notarized. Links to state-specific forms can be found on the websites of various organizations, like the American Bar Association, AARP and the National Hospice and Palliative Care Organization. Learn more in the Resources section.

Once these forms are completed, review them with family or other trusted individuals, as well as your health care team. Keep them in an accessible place and make sure your doctor and others involved in making decisions for your care have a copy. Here's more on each of these documents.

Living will

This legal document spells out what medical treatments you want and don't want to be used to keep you alive. It may also include preferences for decisions like pain management and organ donation. A living will only goes into effect if you're at the end of life.

Whether you want CPR if your heart stops beating, whether you want a machine to keep you breathing and whether you want a tube used to feed you if you can no longer eat are examples of decisions you would spell out in a living will. If you'd like your body to be donated to science for further study, you can specify that in a living will.

Power of attorney

You learned earlier that this legal document gives

PALLIATIVE CARE VS. HOSPICE CARE

Palliative care and hospice care are two terms you'll likely hear. They serve different needs.

Palliative care focuses on providing relief from pain and other symptoms of a serious illness. This type of care isn't just for people who may die soon. It can be offered to people of any age who have a serious or life-threatening illness, no matter the diagnosis or stage of disease. Improving quality of life for people living with dementia and for their families is the goal of palliative care. This form of care is offered alongside other treatments to provide an extra layer of support.

Hospice care is for people who are nearing the end of life. Services are focused on making a person who is terminally ill comfortable. These services reduce pain someone you choose the power to make decisions for you if you're unable to do so. A living will and power of attorney are documents that ensure a person's wishes are respected. However, a power of attorney document is more flexible because the person who is named in the document can make decisions about care that a living will may not address.

A person selected to fill this role should be someone trustworthy who's comfortable talking about medical care and end-of-life issues. It's important to choose an individual who can voice your preferences to your health care team and loved ones. This person shouldn't be your doctor or another member of your health care team.

and address physical, psychological, social and spiritual needs. Hospice care also offers counseling, respite care and practical support to families.

The focus of hospice care is to support the highest quality of life possible for whatever time remains. Hospice care is for a terminally ill person who's expected to have six months or less to live, but it can be provided for as long as the person's doctor and hospice care team certify that the condition remains life-limiting.

Most hospice care is provided at home, with a family member typically serving as the primary caregiver. However, hospice care is also available at hospitals, nursing homes, assisted living facilities and dedicated hospice facilities.

DEMENTIA'S EFFECTS AT THE END OF LIFE

Dementia is a syndrome that causes memory, thinking, behavior and the ability to perform everyday activities to worsen over time. Because people often live with Alzheimer's disease and related dementias for years, it can be hard to think of them as terminal conditions, but they do ultimately lead to death.

It's impossible to predict how quickly dementia will progress, and the end-of-life experience is different for every person. This can make it hard to know when someone is experiencing the symptoms of late-stage dementia. Here are several common signs and symptoms of dementia at the end of life:

- Inability to move around, walk or sit.
- Inability to speak or make oneself understood.
- Inability to perform all or most activities of daily living without help, including bathing, grooming and going to the bathroom.
- Loss of appetite, difficulty swallowing and other eating problems.
- Changes in breathing, often near the end of life, including shortness of breath (dyspnea).
- Excessive sleepiness.
- Seizures and frequent infections, especially pneumonia.
- Restlessness.

Making decisions for someone with dementia

It can be challenging and overwhelming to have to make medical decisions for someone else. In the best circumstances, you'll have written documents that spell out the person's wishes. However, even when you have written documents, decisions aren't always clear. In these situations, it can help to put yourself in the place of the person who's dying. The other approach is to decide what's in the best interest of the person who's dying, given the circumstances and what you know about the person. In these situations, even if one family member is named as the decision-maker, it's a good idea to include the whole family and other trusted individuals in the decision-making process.

Here are some of the medical decisions you may face with advanced dementia.

Feeding tubes

Tube feeding is sometimes suggested if a person has a hard time eating or swallowing — for example, after a stroke. Tube feeding generally isn't recommended for people with dementia even though trouble swallowing may develop in late stages. Tube feeding hasn't been proved to benefit or extend life for people with dementia, and it can lead to infections and cause discomfort.

Before making a decision about feeding tubes, it's best to talk with the health care team about specific plans for their use.

Antibiotics

Antibiotics may be prescribed for common infections. However, they may not improve the person's condition. Again, it's best to weigh the pros and cons of using antibiotics with health care professionals, should the need arise.

Intravenous (IV) hydration

IV hydration is used to give a person liquid through a needle in a vein. Dehydration is part of the dying process; it allows for a more comfortable death over a period of days. IV hydration can cause uncomfortable fluid retention and swelling and draw out the dying process for weeks, which may put a burden on the person who's dying. If IV hydration is considered, it's best if it's used for a limited time period for specific goals — and only if the family and health care team agree that it's best for the person with dementia.

Cardiopulmonary resuscitation (CPR)

CPR is an emergency treatment used to restore a person's heartbeat or breathing if it stops. Many experts do not recommend CPR for people who are terminally ill, and people faced with a terminal illness who can speak for themselves often don't want CPR if their heart or breathing stops. Do not resuscitate (DNR) and do not attempt resuscitation (DNAR) orders tell the health care team not to perform CPR if the person's breathing or heartbeat stops.

Regardless of the options chosen, it's important to continue to maintain the person's dignity and privacy. Advice from a doctor, other specialists and members of a hospice team are important.

OFFERING PERSON-CENTERED CARE

For people with dementia and care partners alike, care at the end of life involves meeting a variety of physical, emotional, social, spiritual and practical needs. For people with dementia, research suggests that the most important facets of a good end-of-life experience are physical, pain-free comfort; emotional and spiritual well-being; family involvement; and a peaceful environment.

Emotional support, for example, may be as simple as a gentle, reassuring touch. It meets a need to feel respected, a need to be with others, a need to feel understood and reassured, and a need to feel loved. Being treated as a person who is still aware of the world is vital.

Connection is critical. It's not only still possible for those with dementia at the end of life, but also essential. Your caring attention and presence are among the most important things you can give someone who's dying. Communication provides stimulation and can help the person with dementia feel reassured and included. Your tone of voice, body language and facial expressions are forms of nonverbal communication that can still be understood by the person with dementia and allow you to connect.

Research shows that at the end of life, a person continues to connect to the world mostly through the senses. This makes touch, sound, sight, taste and smell all powerful ways to connect with a person at the end of life and provide comfort at the same time. Bring in a beloved item for the person to hold, play the person's favorite music, rub lotion with the person's favorite scent on the skin, brush the person's hair or read something aloud that has meaning to the person, like certain religious passages.

Use what you know about the person, including hobbies and interests from the past. Photos, treasured objects and memorabilia can all be helpful in maintaining a connection.

PROVIDING COMFORT AT THE END OF LIFE

Many strategies can help someone with dementia have a dignified death. For someone who's no longer eating or drinking, for example, it can help to keep a person's mouth moist with ice chips or a sponge. Applying lip balm or petroleum jelly to the lips also can provide relief.

Other ways to provide comfort at the end of life include placing pillows behind the person's head to help with labored breathing. Incontinence pads or a catheter helps keep a person with loss of bladder control dry and clean. For cold hands and feet, turning up the heat and providing warm blankets can offer additional comfort.

While not everyone experiences pain when dying, many people do. With dementia, many people aren't prescribed enough pain relief simply because they may not be able to communicate that they're in pain. Pain medications offer another opportunity to improve the end-of-life experience for people with dementia. Experts believe that care for someone who is dying should focus on relieving pain. Pain is easier to prevent than relieve,

SIGNS OF PAIN

A variety of signs can signal discomfort in a person with dementia at the end of life, including the following:
- Agitation.
- Increased confusion or lack of responsiveness.
- Yelling or calling out.
- Grimacing or teeth grinding.
- Scratching or picking at skin or other body parts.
- Excessive sweating.
- Drooling.
- Striking out or other physical gestures of distress.

and overwhelming pain is hard to manage. For those who can't verbally communicate, direct observation of the loved one can help identify pain and pain behaviors.

You may wonder if your loved one is aware of what's going on in this last stage of illness. Although the body and mind are in the process of shutting down, a person with dementia still may be aware of your presence, your care and your affection.

COPING WITH DEATH

When a person with dementia dies, it's common for a care partner to experience many emotions. Loss, depression, anxiety, guilt, frustration and hopelessness are all examples. Likely, these feelings are present even before the person with dementia dies. Nevertheless, emotions near the end of life are often intense, even for care partners who have anticipated and prepared for the death of their loved one. Here are some of the experiences families face after the death of a loved one.

Grief

While grief happens at the end of life, it's also common throughout the dementia process.

Grief can be defined as the process of adjusting to loss. While the grieving process is a gradual one, grief brings powerfully intense feelings and emotions.

The process of allowing yourself to grieve brings about emotional healing and helps you to adjust to a new life situation. Use these recommendations to help support the grieving process:

- Don't try to rush through the grieving process. Over time, you may feel more relief from your grief and less consumed by it. Be gentle with yourself during this time.
- Practice good self-care. Focus on your nutrition, physical activity and sleep.
- Be open with others about what you're experiencing. Your family and friends may avoid the topic, so giving them permission to open up and talk about the loss with you may be helpful.
- Avoid making major decisions for at least a year. This is a period of time when you may still feel unsettled and in shock.
- Follow your usual routine as much as possible, but let others help you with daily tasks. People will want to help you, but they may not know how.
- Acknowledge your emotions. The idea isn't to get caught up in negative or unpleasant feelings but to see that what you're experiencing is OK. Accepting emotions helps to lessen their harsh quality and intensity.
- Reduce any guilt you may feel by trying to keep a realistic view of your past actions and present emotions. Don't focus on what you wish could have been better or what could have been done differently. Believe that you did the best you could and that what you did was enough.

Relief

Some families and care partners experience a feeling of relief — and it's often uncomfortable. It can catch you off guard and feel overwhelming. You may feel guilty when you experience relief.

It's important to know that feeling a sense of relief is natural. In fact, in one study, nearly three-quarters of family caregivers say they felt relieved when an individual with dementia died.

Feeling relief doesn't mean you didn't care about the person with dementia. Instead, relief is a natural response to knowing that the person with dementia is no longer suffering — and that you no longer have to watch someone you care about live with the losses associated with dementia.You may also feel relief because the strain and intensity of being a care partner is lifted. The ability to return to roles you had before becoming a care partner can also bring about feelings of relief.

Feelings of relief are not only natural but also helpful. Some research shows that feelings of relief can actually help care partners grieve more effectively and adjust to life after the person with dementia has died. This is especially true for care partners who felt relatively prepared for the person's death ahead of time.

Loss of identity

For many, the caregiving role lasts several years or much longer, so when the death of their loved one occurs, life can change drastically. There can be an intense feeling of losing both the person and part of who you had become in the caregiving role. Former care partners not only grieve their loved one but also may grieve the loss of the caregiving role. Care partners may find themselves questioning their identity, asking themselves, *Who am I now? Where do I go from here? How do I fill my days and find a sense of purpose?*

In one study, care partners described the post-caregiving phase as a process of learning to live again.

Accustomed to days filled with caregiving responsibilities, care partners recalled not knowing how to proceed with life as they grappled with how to use their free time. Some said they had trouble giving up their role as a care partner after years of identifying with this role.

It's important for care partners to give themselves the space, time and resources they need to adjust to yet another new reality. It's helpful to acknowledge this shift in life and the feelings it may evoke. A care partner may find it therapeutic to write in a journal or share feelings with others in a support group.

As you spend time grieving, healing and adjusting, remember that you and family caregivers like you are the backbone of our health care system. Even if you feel you could have done better, know that what you did is love.

Resources

AARP
www.aarp.org

Administration For Community Living
https://acl.gov

ADVANCE DIRECTIVE FORMS
From AARP
www.aarp.org/caregiving/financial-legal/free-printable-advance-directives

American Bar Association
www.americanbar.org/groups/law_aging/resources/health_care_decision_making/Stateforms

Advancing States
www.advancingstates.org

Agency for Healthcare Research and Quality
www.ahrq.gov

Alzconnected
www.alzconnected.org

Alzheimer's and Related Dementias Education and Referral Center
www.alzheimers.gov

Alzheimer's Association
www.alz.org

Alzheimer's Disease International
www.alz.co.uk

Alzheimer's Foundation of America
https://alzfdn.org

ARCH National Respite Network
https://archrespite.org

Association for Frontotemporal Degeneration
www.theaftd.org

Centers for Medicare & Medicaid Services
www.cms.gov

Certified Financial Planner Board of Standards
www.letsmakeaplan.org/find-a-cfp-professional

Community Resource Finder
www.communityresourcefinder.org

Creutzfeldt-Jakob Disease Foundation, Inc.
https://cjdfoundation.org

CurePSP
www.psp.org

Dementia Action Alliance
https://daanow.org

Dementia Friendly America
www.dfamerica.org/

Department of Veterans Affairs
www.va.gov/find-locations

Eldercare Locator
https://eldercare.acl.gov

Family Caregiver Alliance
www.caregiver.org

Financial and Legal Planning for Caregivers
www.alz.org/help-support/caregiving/financial-legal-planning

Giving Voice Initiative
https://givingvoicechorus.org

House of Memories
www.liverpoolmuseums.org.uk/house-of-memories

I'm Still Here Foundation
www.imstillhere.org

Lewy Body Dementia Association
www.lbda.org

Mayo Clinic
www.MayoClinic.org

Mayo Clinic Connect
https://connect.mayoclinic.org/blog/dementia-hub/

Mayo Clinic's YouTube Channel
www.youtube.com/user/mayoclinic
Keyword search: dementia

Meals on Wheels America
www.mealsonwheelsamerica.org

Medicaid and Medicare
www.medicaid.gov

Medicalert Foundation
www.medicalert.org

National Academy of Elder Law Attorneys
www.naela.org/findlawyer

National Adult Day Services Association
www.nadsa.org

National Association of Area Agencies on Aging
www.usaging.org

National Council on Aging
www.ncoa.org

National Hospice and Palliative Care Organization
www.nhpco.org

National Institute of Neurological Disorders and Stroke
www.ninds.nih.gov

National Institute on Aging
www.nia.nih.gov

National Respite Network and Respite Locator
https://archrespite.org/respitelocator

Parkinson's Foundation
www.parkinson.org

Presence Care Project

www.presencecareproject.com

Social Security Administration

www.ssa.gov

State Health Insurance Assistance Program (SHIP)

www.shiphelp.org

TimeSlips

www.timeslips.org

TrialMatch

www.alz.org/alzheimers-dementia/research_progress/
clinical-trials/about-clinical-trials

World Health Organization

www.who.int/health-topics/dementia

Selected recommended reading

Ahlskog J. Eric. *Dementia With Lewy Bodies and Parkinson's Disease Dementia: Patient, Family, and Clinician Working Together for Better Outcomes*. Oxford University Press, 2014.

Ames Hoblitzelle O. *Ten Thousand Joys & Ten Thousand Sorrows: A Couple's Journey Through Alzheimer's*. Tarcher-Perigee, 2008.

Basting A. *Creative Care: A Revolutionary Approach to Dementia and Elder Care*. HarperOne, 2020.

Boss P. *Loving Someone Who Has Dementia: How to Find Hope While Coping With Stress and Grief*. Jossey-Bass, 2011.

Brackey J. *Creating Moments of Joy Along the Alzheimer's Journey*. Fifth Edition, Purdue University Press, 2016.

Bryden C. *Dancing With Dementia: My Story of Living Positively With Dementia*. Kingsley Publishers, 2005.

Buell Whitworth H., et al. *A Caregiver's Guide to Lewy Body Dementia*. Demos Medical Publishing, 2011.

Chang E., et al. *Living With Dementia: A Practical Guide for Families and Personal Carers.* ACER Press, 2013.

Cornish J. *The Dementia Handbook: How to Provide Dementia Care at Home.* CreateSpace Independent Publishing Platform, 2017.

Kuhn D., et al. *The Art of Dementia Care.* Cengage Learning, 2008.

Manteau-Rao M. *Caring for a Loved One With Dementia: A Mindfulness-Based Guide for Reducing Stress and Making the Best of Your Journey Together.* New Harbinger Publications, 2016.

Neff K., et al. *The Mindful Self-Compassion Workbook: A Proven Way to Accept Yourself, Build Inner Strength, and Thrive.* Guilford Press, 2018.

Pearce N. *Inside Alzheimer's: How to Hear and Honor Connections With a Person Who Has Dementia.* Forrason Press, 2010.

Powell T. *Dementia Reimagined: Building a Life of Joy and Dignity From Beginning to End.* Avery, 2019.

Power G. Allen. *Dementia Beyond Disease: Enhancing Well-Being.* Health Professions Press, 2014.

Snyder L. *Living Your Best With Early-Stage Alzheimer's: An Essential Guide.* Sunrise River Press, 2010.

Towne Jennings J. *Living With Lewy Body Dementia: One Caregiver's Personal, In-Depth Experience.* WestBow Press, 2012.

Zeisel J. *I'm Still Here: A New Philosophy of Alzheimer's Care.* Avery, 2009.

Index

H

I

L

M

S

T

W

MAYO CLINIC | Mayo Clinic Press

Health information you can trust

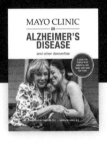

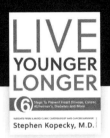

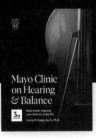

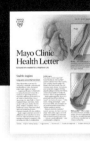

Mayo Clinic on
Alzheimer's Disease
and Other Dementias

Live Younger Longer

Mayo Clinic on
Hearing and Balance,
Third Edition

Mayo Clinic
Health Letter

At Mayo Clinic Press, we believe that knowledge should be shared, especially when it comes to health and medicine. Through printed books and articles, ebooks, audiobooks, podcasts, videos, and more, we provide reliable health information designed to empower individuals to take an active role in their health and well-being.

Our health publications are authored by teams of medical experts, including physicians, nurses, researchers and scientists, and written in language that's easy to understand.

Here is just a sample of some of our other titles:

- Arthritis
- Back and Neck Health
- Mayo Clinic Diet
- Digestive Health
- Prostate Health
- Home Remedies
- Osteoporosis
- Cook Smart, Eat Well
- Family Health
- And many more

Scan to learn more

Discover our full line of publications: MCPress.MayoClinic.org

Mayo Clinic Publications — Reliable. Authoritative. Nonprofit.
Proceeds from the sale of books and subscriptions help support Mayo Clinic programs, including important research and education.